T0358176

Galen's Theory of Black Bile

Studies in Ancient Medicine

Edited by

John Scarborough (*University of Wisconsin-Madison*)
Philip J. van der Eijk (*Humboldt-Universität zu Berlin*)
Ann Ellis Hanson (*Yale University*)
Joseph Ziegler (*University of Haifa*)

VOLUME 51

The titles published in this series are listed at *brill.com/sam*

Galen's Theory of Black Bile

Hippocratic Tradition, Manipulation, Innovation

By

Keith Andrew Stewart

BRILL

LEIDEN | BOSTON

Albrecht Dürer's Melencolia I. Harris Brisbane Dick Fund, 1943. Source:
https://www.metmuseum.org/art/collection/search/336228. Attribution 1.0 Generic (CC BY 1.0)

Library of Congress Cataloging-in-Publication Data

Names: Stewart, Keith Andrew, author.
Title: Galen's theory of black bile : Hippocratic tradition, manipulation,
    innovation / By Keith Andrew Stewart.
Description: Leiden ; Boston : Brill, [2018] | Series: Studies in ancient medicine,
    ISSN 0925-1421 ; volume 51 | Includes bibliographical references and index.
Identifiers: LCCN 2018039970 (print) | LCCN 2018041336 (ebook) |
    ISBN 9789004382794 (ebook) | ISBN 9789004382787 (hardback : alk. paper)
Subjects: LCSH: Galen. | Medicine, Greek and Roman. | Body fluids.
Classification: LCC PA3997 (ebook) | LCC PA3997 .S74 2018 (print) |
    DDC 610.1–dc23
LC record available at https://lccn.loc.gov/2018039970

Typeface for the Latin, Greek, and Cyrillic scripts: "Brill". See and download: brill.com/brill-typeface.

ISSN 0925-1421
ISBN 978-90-04-38278-7 (hardback)
ISBN 978-90-04-38279-4 (e-book)

To Katherine,
Alexander and Reggie

∵

Contents

Acknowledgements

I would like to thank John Wilkins and David Leith for their excellent and patient supervision of my PhD thesis (University of Exeter, 2017), on which this manuscript is based. I would like also to thank both David Braund and Matthew Wright for their support as supervisors at the beginning and end of the PhD. I am very grateful to the Arts and Humanities Research Council for funding three years of my PhD, without this funding I would not have been able to undertake this research. I would also like to thank the Brill referee and Philip van der Eijk for their helpful suggestions and comments. Finally, I want to thank my wife Katherine for her continued love and support to me while I worked on the research for the PhD and this manuscript.

Introduction

The concept of black bile as a substance responsible for health and disease is an interesting topic in ancient medicine. The origin of black bile appears to have originated towards the end of the fifth century BCE, when it was defined as a fundamental substance in the body, alongside blood, phlegm and yellow bile in the Hippocratic *On the Nature of Man*. But, apart from this one treatise, black bile was regarded mostly as a type of waste product or was completely ignored in the medical theories of many physicians and philosophers. Black bile might have remained a fairly insignificant substance in medical writing, if it was not for Galen's reference to the superiority of the four-humour system in *On the Nature of Man*, which raised the status of black bile as an important substance for the explanation of health and disease in the body. It is easy to understand why Galen would use blood, phlegm and yellow bile as fundamental substances in his theory of health and disease, as all three were considered by many physicians and philosophers to be essential for understanding how health and disease occur in the body. However, black bile did not seem to be as highly regarded in medicine and so Galen needed to defend the use of this humour in his medical writing. Therefore, out of these four humours, black bile represents the greatest challenge for Galen, as he attempts to explain how this substance is an essential humour that keeps the body healthy, but also is the cause of the most deadly diseases. In addition, Galen's justification of the very existence of black bile provides an excellent insight into his polemical strategy for the refutation of the theories of his rivals, such as Erasistratus and Asclepiades.

There has been relatively little work done on Galen's writing on black bile across the large number of extant texts in the Galenic corpus.[1] The general view

---

1 One of the earliest and most influential works of modern scholarship on Galen's characterisation of black bile is Schöner's study of humoral theory in the 1960s. Schöner attempts to trace the presence of blood, phlegm, yellow bile and black bile in the work of the most important authorities on aetiology from the time of Hippocrates to that of Galen and afterwards. There is a general emphasis on Galen's presentation of black bile as being a development from the four-humour system of the Hippocratic *On the Nature of Man*. Therefore, black bile is shown to be one of four humours of the body and has its own set of corresponding qualities and properties. Schöner summarises Galen's characterisation of black bile as being sharp and sour in flavour, 'cold and dry' in quality, and is associated with the cosmic 'element' earth, the spleen in the body, the season of autumn, the mature stage of life and the quartan fever. He suggests that Galen has gone beyond the four-humour system of *On the Nature of Man* by drawing upon a wider range of philosophical and medical theories. However, he does not

is that Galen adopted the four-humour system found in the Hippocratic *On the Nature of Man* and then developed his own interpretation of this humoral theory. Therefore, in modern scholarship any mention of black bile tends to be within the context of the other three humours (blood, phlegm and yellow bile) in Galen's version of the four-humour system. For example, Vivian Nutton explains that by Galen's time in the second century CE, the four-humour theory found in *On the Nature of Man* was considered to be Hippocratic and that Galen was in no doubt that this was the theory proposed by the great Hippocrates, rather than by one of his followers.[2] Klibansky, Panofsky and Saxl provide a more focused view of Galen's writing on black bile, as they discuss the case of melancholy illness that Galen associates with issues concerning black bile in the body. Importantly we find reference to Galen's distinction between different types of 'black bile', as they refer to Galen's use of the term 'melancholic humour'. This substance is identified as being one of the four humours, but is different from the black bile that thickens and chills the blood. However, there is no further analysis about what this means to Galen's overall humoral theory and how the 'melancholic humour' is used by Galen more generally in his other treatises.[3] At a similar time in the 1960s, Flashar also analysed the material on melancholy found in Galen's *On Affected Parts* and found that Galen had proposed three ways that melancholy could be produced from black bile. The first cause is where black bile is generated from the blood in the whole body. The second process is when black bilious blood can be found only in the brain. Thirdly, melancholy is caused from the generation of gas in the stomach.[4] Again, Flashar is writing primarily on melancholy. However, there is no

---

provide any analysis of exactly which sources Galen has used and the reasons for the different presentations of black bile in Galen's writing. See Schöner, 1964: 86–93.

2   Nutton, 2005: 116.

3   This characterisation of black bile is based on Galen's *On Affected Parts*, which they use to present Galen's theory of black bile on the basis of two distinct types. One is a natural black bile that is thick and cold, which, as one of the four humours, can only cause harm in large quantities. The other type is 'diseased' black bile that is not one of the four humours and is produced from the combustion of yellow bile. This kind of black bile always causes disease in the body. See Klibansky, Panofsky, and Saxl, 1964: 53.

4   Flashar does not believe that Galen has gone beyond the ideas contained in the Hippocratic Corpus or the Peripatetic works in his writing on melancholy. He points out that Galen refers to an association between black bile and a psychological condition. But Flashar does not regard this as a fully developed doctrine relating to the one of the four temperaments, as at this stage there has been no formal systematic naming of melancholic, choleric, sanguine and phlegmatic temperaments to define a set of psychological conditions. In addition, the later characterisation of the four temperaments differs from Galen's associations of psychological character with the four humours. See Flashar, 1966: 105–109.

attempt to see how this analysis of Galen's writing can be used to further our understanding of black bile in his other treatises. We can find more extensive analysis of Galen's writing on black bile and the diseases caused by this humour in Siegel's 1968 book *Galen's System of Physiology and Medicine*. Siegel investigates Galen's writing on black bile from several treatises and provides information on the key properties of this humour in relation to Galen's view on how it can cause different types of illness, such as diseases of the spleen, anthrax, cancer and melancholy. However, again we find that Siegel tends to generalise Galen's characterisation of black bile, following Schöner's earlier work. There is more detailed analysis that includes some assessment of the information relating to the way that Galen describes black bile, such as the comparison between black bile and the sediment found in wine. But this analysis does not explain why Galen has developed his theory of black bile in different ways in some of his treatises and the implications of these differences. Siegel points out some of the apparent inconsistencies created by the presence of different types of black bile. However, he does not fully investigate the possible reasons, such as the context of the particular argument, which might resolve some of these issues.[5]

If we move forward to more recent studies, there are some more general references to Galen's use of black bile to explain health and disease in the body, such as Langholf's assertion that Galen circumstantially proved the existence of black bile as a distinct substance with reference to the function of the spleen. Here, Langholf uses the ideas contained in Galen's *On Black Bile* as his evidence.[6] This view is reinforced by Grant in his 2000 translation of *On Black Bile*, where he refers to Langholf's analysis, stating that for Galen, black bile did not really exist as an actual substance. Instead, 'black substances', such as dark urine from malaria, are the closest observation of this humour. Grant's view is that the concept of 'black bile' comes from observations of dark or black coloured substances found in the worst kinds of wounds or illness.[7] Mattern provides information on diseases that Galen reports to be caused by black bile, such as elephantiasis, which is due to the accumulation of black bile in the body from certain foods. There is also an association between plague and black bile, as well as breast cancer, epilepsy, and of course melancholy. However, Mattern does not discuss the different types of black bile that Galen writes about in his different treatises. Instead, black bile is portrayed as a single substance that

---

5 Siegel, 1968: 217–322.
6 Langholf, 1990: 46.
7 However, Langholf was mostly working with sources relating to black bile in the Hippocratic Corpus, rather than Galen's treatises. See Grant, 2000: 197 (note 1) and Langholf, 1990: 46–49.

Galen has developed from the Hippocratic Corpus, most notably *On the Nature of Man*.[8] Therefore, so far there is a problem in these more recent studies on Galen's writing about black bile and related diseases, as they do not provide a broad enough explanation of the important details of how and why Galen developed his humoral theory concerning black bile in relation to the Hippocratic Corpus. However, an article by Jacques Jouanna, does attempt to analyse and explain Galen's writing on black bile in more detail.

In a 2009 article, Jouanna investigates the question of the Galenic authenticity of *On Black Bile* and discusses some of the different ways that black bile is characterised in Galen's writing. Passages from *On the Natural Faculties* and *On Black Bile* are compared directly regarding their content on black bile. Jouanna points out that the black bile in *On the Natural Faculties* has the qualities of 'cold and dry', which corresponds to the four-humour system in the Hippocratic *On the Nature of Man*. But he suggests that the black bile in the treatise *On Black Bile* deviates from this model, as it is produced in the presence of hot and dry qualities. Jouanna asserts that the description of black bile in *On the Natural Faculties* is consistent with what he calls the 'founding treatise of *On the Nature of Man*' (*du traité fondateur de La nature de l'homme*), and that this is also Galen's description of black bile in *On the Doctrines of Hippocrates and Plato*.[9] Jouanna explains that the deviation in *On Black Bile* is due 'to a tension in Galen himself' (*d'une tension chez Galien lui-même*), as he attempts to reconcile his characterisation of black bile with *On the Nature of Man* and other sources, from the Hippocratic Corpus and other medical authorities. Jouanna argues that Galen has emphasised the importance of the production of a 'hot' type of black bile at the expense of the traditional conception of black bile as a 'cold and dry' humour, which is found in his other treatises such as *On the Natural Faculties*, *On the Doctrines of Hippocrates and Plato* and the *Commentary on On the Nature of Man*.[10] Jouanna suggests that Galen's characterisation of black bile from the burning of humours is an addition to his theory of the four humours, which he originally developed from the ideas contained in *On the Nature of Man*. Galen did this to incorporate the description of black bile from other Hippocratic sources, which Jouanna identifies as *Airs, Waters and Places* and as material from Rufus of Ephesus.[11] It is the view of Jouanna that Galen

8   Mattern, 2013: 121, 201, 246, 248–249, 251–251; *Meth. Med. Glauc.* 2.12, (XI 140–142 K); *Meth. Med.* 5.12, (X 367 K); *Hipp Aph* 6.23, 6.47 (XVIIIa 35–36, 80 K); Pseudo-Galen, *Cath. Med. Purg.* 1 (XI 344–345 K).
9   Jouanna, 2009: 240–242.
10   Ibid., 2009: 246–247 and 250–252.
11   Hippocratic Corpus, *Aer.*, X (II 50,10–16 L); Rufus of Ephesus, frg. 70 (Pormann) = Ibn Sarā-

was attempting to remain faithful to the four-humour system of *On the Nature of Man* and that he evokes the content of this treatise, even when he is presenting black bile in different ways in *On the Natural Faculties* and *On Black Bile*.

Therefore, we find that there is some acknowledgement that Galen has developed his black bile beyond this Hippocratic treatise, but, apart from Siegel's 1968 book, there has been no major analysis of the different ways that Galen describes the physical appearance and important qualities of black bile in his writing, or any comprehensive investigation of how black bile is produced in the body and its role in the cause of certain types of disease. Therefore, there are two main issues that need addressing regarding Galen's presentation of black bile. Firstly, there is a tendency to either resolve or ignore any inconsistencies in Galen's account of black bile, which over-emphasises the importance of the four-humour system of *On the Nature of Man*. This approach does not take into account other important factors that influence Galen's writing on black bile. Secondly, the current scholarship does not provide enough analysis on Galen's definition and characterisation of the different types of black bile, his strategy to bring together a wide range of sources, and how he uses black bile in different contexts in his treatises. This type of generalisation cannot capture the difference between the various ways that black bile is characterised in the Hippocratic Corpus and the way that Galen uses black bile in his own biological theory. For example, in the history of medicine, the explanation of Galen's development and use of black bile in his theory of health and disease is based on the characterisation of this humour as a development from the ideas contained in the Hippocratic *On the Nature of Man*, but does not discuss the wider range of factors that have influenced Galen's writing on black bile.[12] Therefore,

---

biyūn ibn Ibrāhīm, *Important Chapters on the Medicine of the Masters*, ch. 9, Rufus, *Case Notes* 5. See Jouanna, 2009: 254–255.

12   For example, in Magner's *A History of Medicine*, we find a diagram that neatly summarises the Hippocratic four-humour system, with each humour associated with the four cosmic elements, qualities and temperaments. However, this does not represent the wider content of the Hippocratic Corpus on humoral theory very accurately. We find that black bile is characterised in *On the Nature of Man* and there is no attempt to discuss the different representations of black bile in the other Hippocratic treatises. When the discussion moves on to Galen and the humours, Magner again refers to the type of diagram produced by Schöner in the 1960s, which does not fully represent Galen's use of the humours in his writing. The same kind of diagram is used by Seale to explain how the humours were used by Hippocrates and Galen to present medicine as a model of the relationship between the microcosm and macrocosm in the universe. The problem is compounded further in a summary by Porter, who defines Greek medicine from the time of Hippocrates to Galen in terms of the relationship between the cosmic elements and the four humours. We are told that this is a flexible system that allows the four humours to be associated with the ele-

this analysis does not capture the issues concerning the diversity of the way the humours are presented in the large amount of medical theories produced over several centuries from the fifth century BCE onwards. In addition, there is still an emphasis on the dominance of the theory of the four humours from *On the Nature of Man*. In this way, modern scholarship on Hippocratic and Galenic humoral theory does not provide enough information on the importance of black bile in Galen's theory of disease or the way that he has characterised this humour from a wide range of Hippocratic and other medical and philosophical treatises. In these types of studies on the history of ancient medicine, there is a tendency to generalise the importance of the humours as a group, without any analysis of the role that individual humours play in the explanation of specific types of disease. Therefore, we do not find any reference to the importance of black bile in its own right, as a physiological or pathological substance in the body.

I propose to provide a more comprehensive analysis of the way that Galen defines, characterises and uses black bile in his writing. There are three main areas that I believe need to be addressed further to improve our understanding of how Galen uses black bile in his biological theory of health and disease. The first is to show that the common perception of the dominance of the four-humour system of *On the Nature of Man* is something that has been intentionally presented by Galen, but does not have as much of an influence on his characterisation of black bile, as he would like his audience to believe. Secondly, I will provide a more thorough analysis of the important physical and qualitative properties that Galen uses to define black bile and how this helps him to explain its cause of both health and disease.[13] Thirdly, I am going to investigate

---

ments, qualities, the environment, time of life and the temperaments. See Magner, 1992: 71–73; Seale, 1994: 11 and Porter, 1997: 9, 56–58; 2003: 25–27.

13   I have chosen eight of Galen's treatises for my detailed analysis of his writing on black bile. Firstly, there is the text that he wrote specifically on the black bile humour, called *On Black Bile* (*At. Bil.*). There has been some debate over whether *On Black Bile* can be considered as a genuine work by Galen. However, Jouanna reports that some studies into the Arabic sources on Galen's bibliographical works, *On My Own Books* and *The Order of My Own Books*, provide evidence that this was an authentic treatise by Galen. See Jouanna, 2009: 243–245. *On Black Bile* is important because it contains information, not only on the physical description of black bile and its cause of different types of disease in the body, but it also has some examples of Galen's polemical argument against the work of Erasistratus relating to the importance of understanding the function of black bile in the body. Next, I have chosen the following three treatises: *On the Doctrines of Hippocrates and Plato* (*PHP*), *On the Elements According to Hippocrates* (*Hipp. Elem.*) and *Commentary on On the Nature of Man* (*HNH*). These are important sources, not only for Galen's justification for selection of the four-humour system of *On the Nature of Man*, but also because they con-

how we should understand Galen's presentation of black bile from the way that he manipulates the evidence he uses to support his doxographical and historical presentations, as well as his polemical arguments to refute the theories of his rivals. In addition, I will be analysing how Galen's view of the authenticity of texts in the Hippocratic Corpus may influence the way that he presents black bile in his writing. It is important to investigate the way that Galen defines and uses black bile in relation to the specific context of the whole, or part, of a particular treatise. This is because there is evidence to suggest that apparent inconsistencies in Galen's definition and characterisation of black bile can be explained in relation to the specific argument he is addressing.

---

tain examples of the way that Galen manipulates Hippocratic and other medical sources to show that Hippocrates was the originator of element theory in medicine. The treatises *On the Doctrines of Hippocrates and Plato* and *On the Elements According to Hippocrates* are particularly important for Galen's view that Plato and Aristotle followed the work of Hippocrates on the basis of the qualities, elements and humours for their medical theories. In addition, I have chosen *On the Natural Faculties* (*Nat. Fac.*) and *On the Utility of the Parts* (*UP*) because they provide information on the reasons that Galen gives for his defence of the existence of black bile and its importance in explaining health and disease in the body. Next, I have included *On Mixtures* (*Temp.*), as it describes Galen's theory on how the mixtures of the elemental qualities explain health and disease in the body. In this treatise, the four humours are given a lesser role in the cause of health and disease. However, it contains some useful information on the production of 'black bile' from the action of heat on blood and yellow bile. Galen also says that *On Mixtures* is an essential book to read before moving on to more complicated works, such as *On the Elements According to Hippocrates*. See *Ars. Med.* XXXVII (I 407,8–408,8 K); *Hipp. Elem.* 9.32–35, CMG V 1,2, p. 136,13–23 De Lacy (I 489,2–16 K); *HNH*, I.34, CMG V 9,1, p. 44,3–10 Mewaldt (XV 83,1–10 K). Finally, I have included *On Affected Parts* (*Loc. Aff.*) because it contains information about Galen's writing on the causes of melancholy and other related diseases based on his theory of black bile and other humours. These eight treatises contain key information about Galen's characterisation of black bile based on its physical appearance, key qualities and function for health and disease in the body. They also contain a large amount of material on Galen's biological theory and his use of the black bile humour to explain health and disease in the body. They are important for my analysis, as they contain references to black bile in different forms, as an essential humour for health and a pathogenic substance that causes potentially deadly diseases. These texts also contain examples of Galen's terminology such as 'black bile' (μέλαινα χολή) and 'melancholic humour' (μελαγχολικὸς χυμός), which are important for our understanding of the way that he presents this substance, either as a single concept of a black bile humour, or as three distinct types of black bile. Another important factor is that they provide information on the context of Galen's presentation of black bile in different scenarios, such as agreement between the doctrines of Hippocrates and Plato or refutation of the theories of Erasistratus and Asclepiades. I believe that analysis of the specific context provides essential information to understand the way that Galen characterises black bile. In addition to my main focus on these eight treatises, I will be referring also to a large number of texts from the Galenic Corpus and other important sources.

CHAPTER 1

Galen and the History of Black Bile

1   The Origins of Black Bile and Humoral Theory

An understanding of the way that humoral theory was used in ancient medicine is paramount for an investigation into the importance of black bile as a substance that can explain the cause of health and disease in the body. The term 'humour' comes from the Greek χυμός, which is the essential 'juice' in the body of an animal.[1] However, the term 'humoral theory' should be defined beyond the description of the four fluids found in the Hippocratic *On the Nature of Man*. Instead a more general definition is required, as it is the capacity of these humours or 'juices' to affect the parts of the body that is used to provide an explanation of health and disease in a humoral theory. For example, there is an Aristotelian categorisation that defines the cause of disease on the basis of two distinct types of substance. One is an element (στοιχεῖον), which is a fundamental entity in the body. The other is a residue (περισσώμα) that is produced when disease occurs. This type of waste product is generated by certain processes in the body, such as the action of heat on a substance.[2] This distinction is used in the *Anonymus Londinensis* to provide a doxographical list of the different theories attributed to a set of physicians and philosophers writing on medicine:[3]

---

1   LS&J, page 2013. The use of moistures (ὑγρά) was also important in ancient theories of health and disease. Therefore, there is no reason not to include theories that postulate health and disease on the basis of moistures as being a type of humoral theory. See van der Eijk, 2001: 48.

2   In Aristotle's own theory, health and disease are explained in terms of the four cosmic elements (fire, air, water and earth) and four qualities (hot, cold, wet and dry). Certain humours, such as phlegm, yellow bile and black bile, are considered to be 'residues' of the body that are produced during illness. Therefore, these humours are denied any active power to affect the body in the way that they are in other humoral theories, such as the four-humour system in the Hippocratic *On the Nature of Man*. See Nutton, 2005: 119.

3   The text referred to as the *Anonymus Londinensis* is believed to have been written in the first century CE using Aristotelian sources. There are three sections, the first contains a number of medical definitions and the last section concerns theories of the digestion of food. However, the middle section is of importance here, as it contains a doxography of various theories of disease by a large number of physicians and philosophers. Analysis of this section has revealed that this material is derived either from the work of Aristotle directly or Meno (one of Aristotle's students). See Manetti, 1999: 96–100; Leith, 2015a: 483–484.

© KONINKLIJKE BRILL NV, LEIDEN, 2019 | DOI:10.1163/9789004382794_003

For while some have said that diseases arise because of the residues from nutriment, others hold that they are due to the elements.[4]

It should be noted that this is not a universal theory of the way that substances in the body produce disease. Instead, it is the categorisation used in the *Anonymus Londinensis* to discuss the various different types of aetiological theory available in the medical writing over a long period of time. If the humours are considered as elements, then they represent the fundamental substances in the body and have a physiological and pathological role in the explanation of health and disease. The humours are primary substances in this type of theory and aetiology is determined by three factors: the identification of substances that are elements of the body; the way that these elements cause disease; and the explanation of how various diseases can be produced from these elements. However, if the humours are defined as residues from nutrition, or some other process, they are produced from other substances in the body. In this context the humours are secondary substances and can have physiological and pathological functions as the cause of disease. Disease could occur directly from the residues themselves, or these residues could produce harmful substances that then cause disease. Differences in diseases can be explained by the quantity, quality and location of the residues in the body.[5] Therefore, the humours may be characterised as either elements or residues in the body and this will be useful for understanding how different medical writers use black bile, as an element or a residue, along with the cases where this humour is not included at all in the explanation of health and disease.

There is evidence to suggest that the Hippocratic *On the Nature of Man* is an important treatise for the origins of the characterisation of black bile as a fundamental substance. Jouanna considers *On the Nature of Man* as 'the foundation stone of the history of black bile'. He goes on to claim that the author of this treatise has invented a substance named black bile, associating it with autumn and a particular stage in a person's life.[6] In this way, black bile is raised to be on equal terms to blood, phlegm and yellow bile, all of which have a clearer provenance as fundamental substances in the development of medical theories.[7] For example, blood was thought of as an essential fluid in the body, as much in the ancient world as it is now. This is due to many factors, such

---

4 οἱ μὲν γὰρ εἶπον γίνεσθαι νόσους παρὰ τὰ περισσώματα τὰ γινόμενα ἀπὸ τῆς τροφῆς, οἱ δὲ παρὰ τὰ στοιχεῖα. *Anon. Lond.*, IV,26–28, translation by Jones.

5 Manetti, 1999: 101 and 115.

6 Jouanna, 2012a: 229–230.

7 Müri's opinion is that black bile is a *faute de mieux* and was required to make up the numbers

as the flow of blood from wounds and the presence of blood in bodily fluids during severe illness.[8] Then there is phlegm which is also a substance that can affect health. In the *Iliad*, the goddess Hera stirs up a storm from the sea, which carries bad phlegm (φλέγμα κακόν) that burns up heads and armour.[9] Further to this, bile can also be found in early Greek literature, such as the *Iliad*. For example, Achilles in a rage says that his mother nourished him on bile (χόλος) instead of milk and this bile causes him to be irrational with anger.[10] This type of association between bile and irrational rage is also present within the Hippocratic Corpus. For example, in *The Sacred Disease* heat from bile can cause a corruption of the brain, which makes a person mad, noisy and restless.[11] We can also find the use of bile outside the medical texts, such as a reference to bile in Thucydides, which he uses in his description of the plague of Athens.[12] In this way, we can see that blood, phlegm and bile have had a long tradition in the description of diseases and wounds in early poetic sources all the way down to the writing of the histories in the fifth century BCE. But in the case of black bile, it seems that there is an absence of material on this humour in ancient literature before the mid fifth century BCE.[13]

---

to four to coincide with other phenomena, such as the four seasons and the paired qualities. See Müri, 1953: 27–28.

8   In the writings of Empedocles, blood is very important in the body, not only for reproduction and the growth and development of the embryo, but also because it is the substance in which all four 'roots' are perfectly mixed and, at the location of the heart, it is the agent of thought. Frg. 115 (Graham, 163) = Stobaeus, 1.49.53 (DK 31 B105) and frg. 117 (Graham, 168) = Theophrastus, *On the Senses*, 1,10 (DK 31 A86). See Lonie, 1981: 293.

9   Homer, *Il.* 21.334–337. This is a rare occurrence of phlegm in early Greek literature and it has been suggested by Craik that this may be an early analogy between phlegm being a moving fluid in the body and the deadly rush of water from the sea. However, Lonie does not believe that Homer is describing phlegm as a proper humoral substance and suggests that the first time phlegm is presented as a humour is in Herodotus, who says that the Libyans cauterise the heads and temples of their children to prevent phlegm from flowing down from the head. Herodotus, IV.187; cf. Hippocratic Corpus, *Morb. IV*, IV (XXXV L) (VII 548,11–550,16 L). See Craik, 1998: 99–100 and Lonie, 1981: 277.

10   Homer, *Il.* 16.240 ff.

11   *Morb. Sacr.* XVIII (XV L) (VI 388,12–17 L).

12   Thucydides, II.49.3. Demont suggests that Thucydides understood some aspects of Hippocratic medicine, as he includes a reference to the vomiting of different kinds of bile, which provides a descriptive account for his readers, as well as being consistent with parts of the medical texts at this time, such as what we find in some of the treatises from the Hippocratic Corpus. Therefore, Thucydides aims to provide the proper medical details he requires in order to create a convincing and informative narrative for his readers. See Lonie 1981: 333; Jouanna, 2001: 294 (note 1) and Demont, 2005: 275–276.

13   The general consensus is that *On the Nature of Man* was written sometime in the last few decades of the fifth century BCE. See Craik, 2015: 212.

One of the earliest sources for black bile comes from the Hippocratic *On the Nature of Man*, where it is characterised as a fundamental substance in the body, alongside the other three humours. Here we find black bile described as 'cold and dry', predominant in autumn, associated with ages between 25 and 42 and as the cause of quartan fever. Pain and disease occur when there is more or less black bile than the proper quantity in the mixture, or when it becomes separated from the other humours.[14] However, black bile can be found in many other treatises in the Hippocratic Corpus. For example, in *On Places in Man* there is the following statement about severe wounding of the body:

> Mortal wounds: if it is any kind of a severe one and besides the wounded person vomits black bile, he dies.[15]

Craik argues against an association between this black bile substance in *On Places in Man* and *On the Nature of Man*. Her view is that bile has become black and has transformed into a pathogenic substance, which is then observed as 'black bile' in the vomit.[16] There is no actual explicit statement by the author of *On Places in Man* that bile is changed into black bile by some kind of process in the body. Instead, we are left with black bile appearing in the vomit of someone who has received a mortal wound to the body. The passage quoted above is the only reference to black bile (χολὴ μέλαινα), and we find that this substance is not given the same status as blood, phlegm and bile in this treatise. Therefore, we can say that this is a very different characterisation of black bile than we find in *On the Nature of Man*, as in *On Places in Man*, black bile is being described as a residue produced during the extreme wounding of the body. Another example is the use of black bile as an indicator of specific types of disease. This is found in *Epidemics VI*, where a black tongue indicates the presence of too much black bile in the body that could lead to illness.[17] In other Hippocratic texts, we

---

14   *Nat. Hom.* 4–5; 7 and 15 CMG I 1,3, pp. 172,13–176,1; 182,4–186,12 and 202,10–204,21 Jouanna (VI 38,19–40,17; 46,9–50,13 and 66,10–68,16 L).

15   θανάσιμα τρώματα· ἐφ' ᾧ ἄν τινι κακῶς ἔχοντι χολὴν μέλαιναν ἀπεμέσῃ, ἀποθνῄσκει ὁ τὸ τρῶμα ἔχων. *Loc. Hom.* XXXIII (VI 324,17–18 L), adapted from a translation by Potter.

16   Craik, 1998: 189.

17   *Epid. VI*, v.8 (V 318,5–8 L). See Schöner, 1964: 24–25. It is interesting that the author of *Epidemics VI* uses blood, phlegm, yellow bile and black bile here to demonstrate that different colours of the tongue can be linked to the presence of excessive amounts of these four substances. It is rare to find these four humours being discussed together like this in the Hippocratic Corpus outside *On the Nature of Man*. There is a similar case with diseases of the spleen associated with blood, phlegm, yellow bile and black bile in *Int.* (XXX–XXXIV,

find that black bile is associated with different types of disease. In *Aphorisms*, dysentery that begins with black bile is reported to result in death, and in *On Diseases I*, black bile is said to be the cause of paralysis.[18] There are many other examples in treatises such as *Aphorisms, Epidemics I–VII, Regimen in Acute Diseases, On Internal Affections, On Affections, Koan Prognoses, On Diseases I– III* and *On Diseases of Women II*.[19] What we find is that there are differences between the Hippocratic treatises, with the black bile of *On the Nature of Man* being described as a distinct substance. This is different from what is presented generally as a harmful substance named 'black bile' in other treatises from the Hippocratic Corpus. In addition, there are many Hippocratic texts that refer to blood, phlegm and bile, but not to black bile. This is the case for treatises such as *Prognostic, On the Sacred Disease, On Nutriment* and *On Humours*. When it comes to the illness known as 'melancholy', Jouanna suggests that the Hippocratic treatise, *Airs, Waters and Places*, is the earliest place in Greek literature to describe this disease in the context of the environment and the climate.[20] In other Hippocratic works, such as *Aphorisms*, we have melancholy being characterised in relation to emotional and physical problems.[21] However, there is no clear or consistent development of a theory of melancholy in the Hippocratic Corpus.

There are more examples of the use of black bile within different types of medical theory in the *Anonymus Londinensis*. For example, Dexippus of Cos defines phlegm and bile as the residues of nutriment. These waste products can undergo changes through excess heat or cold to produce white phlegm (λευκὸν φλέγμα) and black bile (μέλαινα χολή). In this humoral theory, phlegm and bile are physiological humours, which can cause disease when they are inhibited in some way in the body. Further to this, the alteration of phlegm and bile produce pathological humours, such as white phlegm and black bile, which are harmful to the body and cause disease.[22] Then there is Menecrates, who postulates that the body is made up of four elements, two that are hot (blood and bile) and two that are cold (breath and phlegm). When these elements are in

---

VII 244,6–252,16 L). In these two cases there is no other content in the texts to suggest that these authors were using the four-humour system of *On the Nature of Man*.

18   *Aph.* IV.24 (IV 510,9–10 L); *Morb. I*, III (VI 144,15–16 L). See Schöner, 1964: 43.
19   For more information on the black bile content of all of these treatises, see chapter 2, section 3 below.
20   *Aer.* X (II 50,6–16 L). See Müri, 1953: 29; Schöner, 1964: 50–51; Jouanna, 2012a: 232.
21   *Aph.* VI.23 (IV 568,11–12 L). See Jouanna, 2012a: 234–235.
22   *Anon. Lond.*, XII,8–36. Large parts of the text are missing at this point and so it is difficult to understand the full meaning of Dexippus' theory from information about the changes to phlegm and bile and any association with blood. See Manetti, 1999: 112.

harmony, the body is healthy, otherwise disease can develop. The changes that occur can produce red bile (πυρρά χολή) or black bile (μέλαινα χολή). Therefore, we have the humours, blood, phlegm and bile, as elements that produce pathological humours such as red bile and black bile. The various types of disease are explained by the movement of these physiological and pathological humours to different places in the body.[23] This is in contrast to the theories of other medical writers that do not include black bile. For example, Thrasymachus of Sardis, Philolaus of Croton and Petron of Aegina include blood, phlegm and bile among the residues that are responsible for causing disease in the body, but not black bile.[24]

2 Galen's Doxographical Explanation for the History of Black Bile

When it comes to identifying the framework for Galen's writing on black bile, we find that there is significant emphasis on the black bile from the four-humour system of *On the Nature of Man*, which Galen identifies as the humoral system created by Hippocrates.[25] We can see this from statements in many of Galen's treatises, such as *On the Elements According to Hippocrates*, *Commentary on On the Nature of Man* and *On the Doctrines of Hippocrates and Plato*.[26] Therefore, as black bile is one of these four humours, it has a high status in Galen's medical writing as a fundamental substance to explain health and disease in the body. We find this is the case when Galen discusses the four humours

---

23 *Anon. Lond.*, XIX,18–XX,1. See Schöner, 1964, 75; Huffman, 1993: 294; Manetti, 1999: 117.

24 Thrasymachus of Sardis is otherwise unknown outside of the *Anonymus Londinensis* (XI,43–XII,8). See Schöner, 1964: 65; Huffman, 1993: 293 and 302; Manetti, 1999: 111–112; Nutton, 2004: 52 and 80; 2005: 117–118. For Philolaus, see *Anon. Lond.*, XVIII,8–XIX,1 and Lloyd, 1963: 120; Huffman, 1993: 5–6; 87–89, 291, 297–298 and 301–306; Manetti, 1999: 115–116. For Petron, see *Anon. Lond.*, XX,1–24 and Huffman, 1993: 304.

25 In contrast, the *Anonymus Londinensis* (XIX,2–18) presents Hippocrates as postulating the cause of disease from gases in the body, which can be produced from the ingestion of food that is excessive, too varied or difficult to digest. The doxography here is not from just one Hippocratic text and Manetti suggests that it is based on the Hippocratic use of a term for 'food' (πρόσαρμα), which is otherwise not used in the *Anonymus Londinensis*. The author of *On the Nature of Man* is identified as Polybos, following Aristotle's view of authorship. See Manetti, 1999: 103–106 and 116–117. I will discuss the issues regarding the authorship of different parts of *On the Nature of Man* in detail later, see chapter 2, section 3 below.

26 *Hipp. Elem.* 8.12–9.3; 11.1–3, CMG V 1,2, pp. 126,5–26; 140,15–142,1 De Lacy (I 479,16–481,10; 494,1–11 K); *HNH*, I.19, CMG V 9,1, pp. 32,10–33,21 Mewaldt (XV 59,1–61,12 K); *PHP*, VIII.4.1–7, CMG 4,1,2, pp. 498,17–500,2 De Lacy (V 671,11–673,2 K).

and refers to each of them as 'elements' of the body.[27] In *On the Therapeutic Method*, Galen sets out what he regards as the history of the development of the elemental qualities, hot, cold, dry and wet:

> But if we were to empanel the philosophers of the Stoa and entrust the vote to them too, as a result of the doctrines they themselves affirm, they would crown Hippocrates. For it was Hippocrates who first of all introduced the doctrine of the Hot, the Cold, the Dry, and the Wet; later Aristotle gave a demonstration of it. Chrysippus and his followers took it over ready-made, and did not indulge in futile strife, ... Thus in the eyes of Plato, the Peripatetics, and the Stoics, Hippocratic natural science wins the day ... But if we pass over Plato, Aristotle, and Chrysippus and their followers as being unversed in this matter, we won't find anyone else who is.[28]

In this passage, we can see that Galen names Plato, Aristotle, Chrysippus and their followers as those who have correctly followed Hippocrates' theory of the elemental qualities.[29] However, if we investigate the specific details of the theories relating to the occurrence of health and disease in the human body, we find that Galen is not always in complete agreement with Plato, Aristotle or the Stoics.[30]

---

27   Galen refers to these fundamental substances, collectively as the 'four humours' (τεσσάροι χύμοι). For example, see *PHP*, VIII.4.4, CMG V 4,1,2, 498,26–28 De Lacy (V 672,5–8 K). But this is not generally the terminology used in *On the Nature of Man*. There is only one reference to the term 'humour' in the fifteenth section of *Nat. Hom*. (15, CMG I 1,3, p. 204,12–14 Jouanna (VI 68,6–8 L)), where black bile is described as the most sticky of the humours (χύμοι). Interestingly, this is in the part of *On the Nature of Man* that Galen considers as inauthentic. For more information, see chapter 2, section 3 below.

28   εἰ δὲ τοὺς ἀπὸ τῆς στοᾶς φιλοσόφους εἰς τὸ συνέδριον εἰσαγαγόντες ἐπιτρέψαιμεν καὶ τούτοις τὴν ψῆφον, ἐξ ὧν αὐτοὶ τίθενται δογμάτων, ἐκ τούτων Ἱπποκράτην στεφανώσουσι. τὸ γὰρ θερμὸν καὶ τὸ ψυχρὸν καὶ τὸ ξηρὸν καὶ τὸ ὑγρὸν Ἱπποκράτης μὲν πρῶτος εἰσηγήσατο, μετ' αὐτὸν δ' Ἀριστοτέλης ἀπέδειξεν· ἕτοιμα δ' ἤδη παραλαβόντες οὐκ ἐφιλονείκησαν οἱ περὶ τὸν Χρύσιππον, ... ὥστε καὶ κατὰ Πλάτωνα καὶ κατὰ τοὺς ἐκ τοῦ περιπάτου καὶ κατὰ τοὺς ἐκ τῆς στοᾶς ἡ Ἱπποκράτους νικᾷ φυσιολογία· ... ἀλλ' ἐὰν τοὺς περὶ Πλάτωνα καὶ Ἀριστοτέλη καὶ Χρύσιππον ὡς ἀγυμνάστους ἐν τῇδε παρέλθωμεν, οὐχ εὑρήσομεν ἑτέρους. *MM*, I.2.9–10; 2.11–12; 2.13 (X 15,18–16,5; 17,2–4; 18,4–6 K), translation by Hankinson.

29   Jouanna, 2002b: 256–257.

30   For example, there is influence from Plato in Galen's work on physiology and anatomy, such as his reference to a three-part division of the soul. See Vegetti, 1999a: 342–344 and Singer, 2013: 348–349. On the subject of the human psyche, Galen attacks the Stoic position in *On the Doctrines of Hippocrates and Plato*. However, Galen's view of Stoicism was not always negative. It is true that we can find a large amount of criticism of the Stoics in

Galen adopts a similar system to the Aristotelian concept of three levels of physical substance in his treatise *The Best Doctor is also a Philosopher*. The most fundamental level consists of the 'primary elements' (πρῶτα στοιχεῖα) which mix together to form more substantial matter.[31] Uniform or homogeneous (ὁμοιομερής) substances are the second level of matter and the third level contains the more complex structures, such as the organic (ὀργανικός) parts of the body.[32] In *On the Natural Faculties*, Galen explains the interaction of substances on the basis of capacity or faculty (δύναμις), which defines the attractive, retentive and assimilative nature of fluids, substances and organs in the body.[33] Therefore, when it comes to the language used to write about fundamental matter, Galen has a tendency to select terms that are distinctly

---

On the Doctrines of Hippocrates and Plato and in the eleventh chapter of *The Faculties of the Soul Follow the Mixtures of the Body*. But, on the other hand, there are texts where Galen offers a more positive view of Stoicism. This is the case when he is prepared to bring them onto his side in certain debates, such as supporting his view of the fundamental matter as a mixture of elements against the theory of the atomists. For example, see *PHP*, II.2.4–14, CMG V 4,1,2, pp. 104,3–106,23 De Lacy (V 213,8–216,15 K); *QAM*, 11 (IV 816,8–819,15 K). There is in fact a large amount of commonality between Galen's theory of human psychology and that of the Stoics. Gill suggests that Galen may have been able to improve his writing on human psyche, if he had been more tolerant towards the Stoics. This is because the Stoic theory of the embodied nature of the psyche is more closely aligned to Galen's views than that of Plato's tripartite division, which Galen favours. Therefore, Galen is selective and will sometimes acknowledge the influence of certain philosophers, or philosophical schools, on his writing about different topics. But Galen's use of both medical and philosophical sources is complex, as he does not always tell us that he has been influenced by a particular source. The one common point that Galen makes is that the basis for all this work on elemental theory that applies to the explanation of health and disease began with Hippocrates. See Gill, 2010: 1–7 and 26–27.

31   The primary level is the four cosmic 'elements': fire, air, water and earth. These are in turn formed from four basic qualities: hot, cold, dry and wet, which are more fundamental than other types of quality, such as density or texture. The second level of composition refers to the uniform parts of the body, such as bone and flesh. Finally, the third level is based on the non-uniform parts, which represent the hands or the face, etc. What we find is that Galen has drawn upon this Aristotelian system for his own theory of substances in the human body. But Kupreeva has raised a point about a possible difference between the language used by Galen and Aristotle in their presentation of elemental substances. We find that Galen defines the στοιχεῖα as 'simple substances', which contain the qualities. In contrast, Aristotle refers to 'out of powers' (δυνάμεις), which he defines as the 'simple qualities'. Aristotle, *PA*, II, 646a12–24. See Peck and Forster, 1937; Kupreeva, 2014: 161–162; Leith, 2015a: 462–463.

32   *Opt. Med.* 3 (I 60,1–8 K). See Hankinson, 2008: 210–211. Galen combines Hippocratic physiology with Aristotelian elemental theory. The key texts from Aristotle are: *Parts of Animals*, *On Generation and Corruption* and *Meteorology*. See van der Eijk, 2014: 100–101.

33   *Nat. Fac.* I.4 (II 9,7–10,5 K). See Gill, 2010: 70.

Aristotelian. However, we find that Galen has developed the language further than it appears in its Aristotelian context.[34] This is part of Galen's strategy to present what he considers to be Hippocrates' work in Aristotelian language, which makes it easier for him to associate the work of Hippocrates with that of Aristotle.[35] However, there is a problem with Galen's view that Hippocrates was the first to propose and demonstrate a theory of the elements. This is because there is no evidence for a Hippocratic demonstration of the elements and qualities in the way that we find in the Aristotelian sources, such as *Posterior Analytics*. In fact, Aristotle is relegated by Galen to being someone who has continued the work of Hippocrates on elements by providing some demonstrations of Hippocrates' theoretical framework.[36] But in *On the Natural Faculties*, Galen sees this problem as less important relative to the larger debate between the continuum and atomistic theorists. Gill argues that Galen's adoption of parts of Stoic teleology and elemental theory is justified because it is based on the development of 'high naturalism' against the opposing mechanical explanation, proposed by the atomists.[37] The context here is that Galen needs to draw

---

34   One example is Galen's use of the term 'first substance' (πρώτη οὐσία) in relation to his
      view of what is meant by underlying matter, which is found in a slightly different con-
      text in Aristotle's works. *HNH*, Pref. CMG V 9,1, pp. 3,24–4,5 Mewaldt (XV 3,1–7 K); *Lib. Prop.*
      12 (XIX 45,6 K). See Singer, 2014: 34. Another example, which comes from Galen's *On the
      Elements According to Hippocrates*, contains the terms: 'elements' (στοιχεῖα) and 'first prin-
      ciples' (ἀρχαί), which are traditionally considered to have been defined by Aristotle. But
      Galen has developed these terms beyond what we find in Aristotle's writing, as he uses
      more detailed definitions of both στοιχεῖα and ἀρχαί. *Hipp. Elem.* 6.39, CMG V 1,2, p. 114,21–
      23 De Lacy (I 470,5–7 K); cf. Aristotle, *GC*, II.1, 329a27–33; *PA*, II, 648b9–11. See Hankinson,
      2008: 214; Singer 2014: 33. The terms στοιχεῖα and ἀρχαί are also found in Plato's *Timaeus*,
      where fire, air, water and earth are called principles (ἀρχαί) and are described as elements
      (στοιχεῖα) of the universe, like the letters of the alphabet are the elements of language.
      See Plato, *Ti.* 48b. Galen's application of the term for elements (στοιχεῖα) is particularly
      interesting, as he frequently utilises it in his explanation of the ideas contained in Hip-
      pocratic works, when referring to fundamental substances. For example: see *Hipp. Elem.*
      1.3–4, CMG V 1,2, p. 56,9–14 De Lacy (I 414,3–5 K). However, the term στοιχεῖον is not found in
      the Hippocratic Corpus in the context of a fundamental substance. Instead, there is only
      one instance of the use of στοιχεῖον in the extant Hippocratic Corpus and this refers specif-
      ically to one object as part of a set of a larger set of objects, not to fundamental matter.
      Hippocratic Corpus, *Mul.* III, 230 (VIII 444,4–5 L).

35   Galen's strategy here, as Vegetti points out, is to show that there is a clear association
      between what he considers to be a Hippocratic physiology based on a four-humour sys-
      tem with parts of the Aristotelian and Alexandrian anatomical theories. *Nat. Fac.* I.9 (II 19
      K). See Vegetti, 1999a: 351.

36   *MM*, VII.3 (X 462,18–463,2 K); *Lib. Prop.* 11 (XIX 42,3–7 K). See Hankinson, 2008: 211.

37   *MM*, I.2.10 (X 15,18–16,10 K); *Temp.* I.3 (I 523,4–12 K); *Nat. Fac.* I.2 (II 5,4–16 K). For the mate-
      rial from Stoic theory: Stobaeus, 1.129,2–130,13 (LS 47A); Diogenes Laertius, 7.137 (LS 47B);

upon a wide range of sources to attack his opponents on the complex topic of the nature of fundamental matter and how it helps to explain the cause of health and disease in medicine.

We have seen that one of the most important Hippocratic texts that Galen uses to show evidence that Hippocrates was the originator of an elemental theory is *On the Nature of Man*. For example, in the seventh chapter of this treatise, there is a passage that describes the four qualities (hot, cold, dry and wet) as fundamental to all things in the universe. Galen uses this passage as evidence that Hippocrates had an elemental basis for his theory of the four humours and that when Hippocrates refers to the four qualities, he actually means the four elements (fire, air, water and earth).[38] The importance to Galen of the actual status of fundamental substances, from the use of terms such as 'quality' and 'element', is shown in the dialectical debate about the view of the Pneumatist Athenaeus of Attalia in *On the Elements According to Hippocrates*. In this debate we find that Galen criticises Athenaeus' view that the qualities can exist independently from the substances, in which they are manifest. He ridicules anyone who would differentiate between something that contains 'hot' in an extreme sense and the elemental 'fire'.[39] This is important when Galen refers to black bile as being 'cold' and 'dry' in quality, as we understand Galen's characterisation in relation to the interaction between physical substances, such as the cosmic elements or the humours. This interaction is based on the capacity of the physical substance that has inherent qualities. Therefore, it is the physical

---

Plutarch, *On common conceptions*, 1085c–d (LS 47G); Gal. *PHP*, V.3.8, CMG V 4,1,2, p. 306,23–28 De Lacy (V 447,3–9 K) (LS 47H); Alexander, *On mixture*, 224,14–17, 23–26 (LS 47I); Alexander, *On mixture*, 216,14–218,6 (LS 48C). See Gill, 2010: 75–77. However, Galen's assimilation of Stoic physics is not entirely compatible with his own views, particularly in relation to revisionism (willingness to revise familiar distinctions) and holism (a tendency to analyse the whole, rather than the constituent parts). See Gill, 2010: 77–84. I will be discussing Galen's teleological framework for his biological theory in more detail in chapter 2, section 1 below.

38   In this way, Galen is challenging the Pneumatist view of proximate elements, because their view is that the qualities (hot, cold, dry and wet) are all that are needed in medicine, rather than using the four 'cosmic' elements, fire, air, water and earth. Galen believed that the Pneumatists were dissociating the 'art' of medicine from natural philosophy. Hippocratic Corpus, *Nat. Hom.* 7, CMG I 1,3, pp. 184,16–186,10 Jouanna (VI 48,20–50,9 L); Gal., *HNH*, I.38; I.39, CMG V 9,1, pp. 48,13–25; 49,4–7 Mewaldt (XV 91,12–92,9; 93,1–4 K). See Kupreeva, 2014: 158–160. The direct association between these fundamental substances, allows Galen to develop a biological theory that links the four humours of the body to the four cosmic elements in the universe, which enables him to draw upon the natural philosophy of Plato and Aristotle, as well as the physiology of Hippocrates. Kupreeva, 2014: 161.

39   *Hipp. Elem.* 6.1–30, CMG V 1,2, pp. 102,1–110,7 De Lacy (I 457,5–465,1 K). See Smith, 1979: 87–88; Hankinson, 2008: 215–216.

substance of black bile itself that has the capacity to be 'cold' and 'dry'. This seems to bring Aristotelian theory closer to a concept of qualitative interaction that is similar to the type of theory that was adopted later by the Pneumatists, where the qualities are themselves able to interact, rather than being manifest within the four cosmic elements. However, Galen does not want to criticise Aristotle on the subject of elementary substances, as he is using parts of Aristotle's language and doctrine for his own presentation of this subject. But, he can challenge the Pneumatists' view of elementary qualities instead. In this way, Galen is adapting Aristotelian elemental theory for his own use in *On the Elements According to Hippocrates*. But there is a difference in emphasis between Galenic and Aristotelian elemental theories, where Galen regards the concept of an element as a more robust philosophical notion and, as we have seen above, Aristotle is more reluctant than Galen to view 'elements' as physical substances.[40] Therefore, Galen is able to select what he requires from Aristotelian elemental theory and can ignore parts of it that either he does not agree with, or may contradict his own theory. It also allows Galen to refer to Hippocrates, not Aristotle, as the originator of the theory of elements. In *On the Elements According to Hippocrates* Galen uses ideas contained in the Hippocratic *On the Nature of Man* to claim that Aristotle is really a follower of the natural philosophy developed by Hippocrates. In this way, Galen claims that Aristotle adopted Hippocrates' ideas and methodology, and has demonstrated some parts of Hippocrates' element theory. However, the detail of the theory and language used by Galen comes from Aristotle, not from any Hippocratic source, and so this is a clear example of Galen's manipulation of the source material on elements to distort the history of the development of the theory of elements that he uses in his writing. Therefore, Galen is attempting to show that Hippocrates and Aristotle are in agreement on elemental and humoral theory.

There are examples of a more general argument by Galen that the *On the Nature of Man* humoral theory was more universally adopted by some of the most prominent physicians and philosophers over a period of several centuries. We see this from the following passage in Galen's *On the Doctrines According to Hippocrates and Plato*:

> Not only Plato but also Aristotle, Theophrastus and the other followers of Plato and Aristotle emulated the reasoning of Hippocrates on the humours, as did also the most esteemed ancient physicians, Diocles, Pleistonicus, Mnesitheus, Praxagoras, Phylotimus and Herophilus.[41]

---

40   Kupreeva, 2014: 192–193.
41   οὐ μόνος δὲ Πλάτων, ἀλλὰ καὶ Ἀριστοτέλης καὶ Θεόφραστος οἵ τε ἄλλοι μαθηταὶ Πλάτωνός τε καὶ

This list represents Galen's focus on Rationalism in relation to what he considers as the theory of the humours first proposed by Hippocrates himself.[42] In this way, Galen regards Hippocrates as a Rationalist, just like the physicians Diocles and Mnesitheus.[43] This is not the first time this kind of association had been made, as we find that the first century CE physician Celsus includes Hippocrates and Herophilus among the Rationalist physicians. The Rationalist approach to medicine is, as Pellegrin defines, one which does not consider medicine to be based solely on manifest causes, such as indigestion or sunstroke. Instead, medicine should be based on knowledge about the changes at the level of the basic components of the body, such as tissues or the humours. However, at this level it is not possible to make direct observations, but hidden

---

Ἀριστοτέλους οἳ τὸν περὶ τῶν χυμῶν λόγον ἐζήλωσαν Ἱπποκράτους, ὥσπερ γε καὶ τῶν παλαιῶν ἰατρῶν οἱ δοκιμώτατοι, Διοκλῆς, Πλειστόνικος, Μνησίθεος, Πραξαγόρας, Φυλότιμος, Ἡρόφιλος. *PHP*, VIII.5.24, CMG V 4,1,2, p. 510,1–5 De Lacy (V 684,17–685,4 K), translation by De Lacy. There is a similar listing in *Nat. Fac.* II.8; II.9 (II 117,8–12; 140,15–18 K).

42   This list should not be considered as exhaustive, and so Galen may have selected other authorities for this association with his concept of Hippocratic humoral theory. For example, it is interesting that Galen did not include the first century CE physician, Rufus of Ephesus, in his list of physicians and philosophers that adopted Hippocrates' theory of the humours, as at the beginning of *On Black Bile*, Galen names Rufus as an important source on matters relating to the effect of black bile in the body. See *At. Bil.* 1, CMG V 4,1,1, p. 71,12–14 De Boer (V 105,3–5 K). Rufus was a prolific writer and wrote works on various medical topics, but unfortunately only very little of his work has survived. The humours were an important part of his medicine, but from what we know of his writing, he has based his humoralism in relation to his practice of using therapeutic methods, rather than the type of physiological theory that we find in the Hippocratic *On the Nature of Man* or in Galen's writing. Rufus believed that first a doctor should try to identify disease by external manifestations in order for treatment to be tailored specifically to each patient. See Nutton, 2004: 214–215; Pormann, 2008: 146–147. When it comes to the cause of the melancholy illness, Rufus made a distinction between two types of black bile. The first black bile is less harmful, particularly when it has settled in its mixture with blood. The second type of black bile is more harmful and is produced by the heating of yellow bile. For the reference to the first type of black bile: Rufus of Ephesus, F21 (Pormann) = ar-Rāzī, *Comprehensive Book*. For the more dangerous type of black bile produced from yellow bile: F11 (Pormann) = Aëtius, *Medical Books*, vi. 9. See Pormann, 2008: 5. In addition, Rufus wrote about the association between black bile and the spleen, as melancholy was linked to an illness in the spleen and the treatment involves the purging of the 'burnt' substances in the blood. See Rufus of Ephesus, F66 (Pormann) = Ibn Sarābiyūn ibn Ibrāhīm, *Important Chapters on the Medicine of the Masters*, ch. 9, Rufus, *Case Notes* 1. Therefore, there might be some argument to suggest an affinity between the work of Rufus and the Hippocratic *On the Nature of Man*; but Galen chooses not to list this physician among his most important humoral theorists.

43   Nutton, 2004: 125–126.

causes can be inferred logically from the symptoms observed.[44] It is within this
context that Galen claims that some of the early medical authorities adopted
Hippocrates' four-humour system:

> Pleistonicus, Praxagoras, Philotimus, and their followers, working most
> diligently to the greatest extent on the theory of the humours seem use-
> fully to have determined some parts of the undefined writing by Hip-
> pocrates, some parts they have spoken out falsely.[45]

Here we find that Galen is actually acknowledging that some Hippocratic works
can be brief and lacking in detail. We can see that Galen has made explicit
statements that associate the work of Plato, Aristotle, Theophrastus, Diocles,
Pleistonicus, Mnesitheus, Praxagoras, Phylotimus and Herophilus with what
he considers to be Hippocrates' four-humour system.

This implies that these philosophers and physicians regarded each of the
four humours as elements of the body, which explain the cause of health and
disease. In particular, he is asserting that they consider black bile to exist as a
fundamental substance in the body. However, it is likely that Galen has manip-
ulated the writing on the theory of disease of the physicians and philosophers
that he lists as following the four-humour system of *On the Nature of Man*. There
is not one case where there is clear evidence that any of these authorities had
adopted the system of the four humours. The aetiological theories of Diocles,
Mnesitheus and Herophilus seem at first to offer some evidence for a four-
humour system similar to that found in *On the Nature of Man*. But, in the case
of Herophilus, I am in agreement with the arguments that he did not use the
four-humour system of *On the Nature of Man*.[46] When it comes to Mnesitheus,

---

44   Celsus, *On Medicine*, Pref. 15 and 23. See Pellegrin, 2009: 669–670.

45   οἱ δὲ περὶ Πλειστόνικόν τε καὶ Πραξαγόραν καὶ Φιλότιμον ἐπὶ πλεῖστον ἐξεργασάμενοι τὸν περὶ
      τῶν χυμῶν λόγον ἔνια μέν μοι δοκοῦσι χρησίμως διορίσασθαι τῶν ἀδιορίστως Ἱπποκράτει γεγραμ-
      μένων, ἔνια δὲ καὶ ψευδῶς ἀποφήνασθαι. *At. Bil.* 4, CMG V 4,1,1, p. 71,9–12 De Boer (V 104,9–105,3
      K). The Philotimus named here is the same Phylotimus that was referred to in the passage
      from *On the Doctrines According to Hippocrates and Plato* quoted above. See Grant, 2000:
      197.

46   In general, Galen was impressed with Herophilus' discoveries in anatomy and viewed
      them as confirming parts of what he considered to be Hippocrates' theory on the ben-
      efits of therapeutics. However, Galen criticised Herophilus for ignoring the importance
      of the elemental qualities, hot, cold, dry and wet. Frg. T232 (von Staden) = Galen, *MM*,
      X 309,15–310,8 K; frg. T233 (von Staden) = Galen, *MM*, X 184,8–185,2 K; frg. T234 (von Staden)
      = Celsus, *On Medicine*, III.9; frg. T237 (von Staden) = Galen, *Ven. Sect. Er.* VI (XI 169,2–17 K);
      frg. T238 (von Staden) = Galen, *Ven. Sect. Er.* V (XI 162,18–163,6 K). There has been some
      debate on whether Herophilus can be considered as adopting the four-humour system of

it is impossible to determine his position on the four humours, given the lack of information that we have on his medical theory.[47] It is possible that some of the material that we have on Diocles' writing could support Galen's inclusion of this physician in the adoption and development of the humoral system in *On the Nature of Man*. However, I am inclined to agree with van der Eijk's assessment

---

On the Nature of Man, or that he actually postulated a more generalised theory of disease. In his 1989 study of the work of Herophilus, von Staden argues against Kudlien's view that Herophilus was sceptical about the role of the four humours to explain the cause of disease in the body. Von Staden points out that Kudlien's argument primarily rests on ideas contained in two sources, one is the Pseudo-Galen, *Def. Med.* 149 (XIX 391,1–4 K) and the other is Celsus, *On Medicine*, Pref. 14–15. Kudlien suggests that Herophilus adopted a theory based on moistures, not humours and that this was only in reference to therapeutic treatments. Von Staden counters this argument from the fact that the passage from *Def. Med.* refers to the followers of Herophilus, and that Celsus regarded the terms 'moisture' and 'humour' as interchangeable. See von Staden, 1989: 242–246; cf. Kudlien, 1964a: 7–8 and 1964b: 8. However, Nutton states that there is no clear evidence that Herophilus used the four-humour system of *On the Nature of Man*. See Nutton, 2005: 118–119. According to von Staden the material in Galen's *On the Doctrines of Hippocrates and Plato* and *Diagnosis of Pulses*, along with the Pseudo-Galen *Introduction* and *Commentary on On Nutriment*, provides unambiguous statements that Herophilus attributed health and disease to the four-humour theory of *On the Nature of Man*. PHP, VIII.5.24, CMG 4,1,2, p. 510,1–5 De Lacy (V 684,17–685,4 K); *Dig. Puls.* II.3 (VIII 870,8–18 K); Pseudo-Galen, *Int.* IX (XIV 698,16–699,2 K); *Hipp. Alim.* III.21 (XV 346,8–19 K). See von Staden, 1989: 244–245. In the case of black bile, there are only two sources that refer specifically to this humour. One is from Galen's *Commentary on Aphorisms*, which refers to the Herophilean Bacchius' (along with the Empiricists Heraclides and Zeuxis) reading of an aphorism that associates alvine discharges with black bile. The other comes from the pseudo-Galen *Commentary on On Nutriment*, where there is a claim that Plato is in agreement with Herophilus (among others) in his writing on black bile. *Hipp. Aph.* VII.70, (XVIIIa 186,12–187,3 K); *Hipp. Alim.* III.21 (XV 346,8–19 K). See von Staden, 1989: 83, 244 and 312–313. Neither of these sources can be used as evidence for Herophilus' use of black bile in his theory of disease, as Galen's *Commentary on Aphorisms* refers to Bacchius, not Herophilus and the *Commentary on On Nutriment* just compares Herophilus' view of black bile with that of Plato, which hardly refers to black bile at all. Leith has argued that Herophilus postulated the cause of disease from residues in the body. This is different from Galen's description of the four humours based on the elements. Therefore, it is more likely that Herophilus' aetiology of disease is closer to that of the Aristotelian view relating to the production of residues from natural processes in the body. Leith, 2014: 485. Schöner, 1964: 61; Nutton, 2004: 127–131, 135.

47 Mnesitheus, a mid-fourth century BCE physician, did use both χυμός and χυλός to denote an important fluid in the body. However, there is not enough information from the fragments attributed to the work of Mnesitheus to determine whether he adopted the four-humour system of *On the Nature of Man*, or whether he was using a more general humoral theory to explain health and disease in the body. Frgs. 10–14 B (Bertier). See Nutton, 2004: 125; 2005: 118.

on the unreliability of sources on Diocles' use of the humours such as those in the *Anonymus Bruxellensis*, the *Anonymus Parisinus* and Galen.[48] When it comes to the medical theory of Plato, we can find reference to humours, such

---

48   There is evidence that Diocles postulated his theory of disease on the basis of blood, phlegm, yellow bile and black bile. However, there is some difficulty in obtaining an accurate picture of exactly what he wrote and its relationship to the Hippocratic Corpus. For example, Pliny the Elder describes Diocles as 'second in age and in fame' (secundus aetate famaque) to Hippocrates. Frg. 4 (van der Eijk) = Pliny the Elder, *NH*, XXVI.6. Then, we find that in the *Anonymus Bruxellensis* there is a reference to Diocles as a 'follower of Hippocrates' (sectator Hippocratis) and that 'the Athenians call [him] a younger Hippocrates' (Athenienses iuniorem Hippocratem uocauerunt). Frg. 3 (van der Eijk) = *Anonymus Bruxellensis*, *On the Seed* 2 (p. 209,9–10 Wellmann); frg. 4 (van der Eijk) = Pliny the Elder, *NH*, XXVI.6. See Flashar, 1966: 50; van der Eijk, 2000: vii; Nutton, 2004: 122. However, as van der Eijk points out, the statement about Diocles being a younger Hippocrates needs to be considered within the later context of the division of the medical tradition into separate schools. In this sense Diocles is being associated with Hippocrates within the Rationalist (or Dogmatic) school of medicine. This, as van der Eijk suggests, might be related to the 'lists' that he was drawing upon or to the fact that Diocles' fame had risen so far by this time. See van der Eijk, 2001: 7–9. We also have the possibility of an association between Diocles' writing on humours and the Hippocratic *On the Nature of Man*. In the *Anonymus Bruxellensis*, there is the following quotation attributed to Diocles. Frg. 40 (van der Eijk) = *Anonymus Bruxellensis*, 1–8 (p. 208,1–213,14 Wellmann). However, van der Eijk points out that the authorship of this text is now considered to be uncertain. The references to the four humours are from the second chapter of this text and the form of direct speech implies that this may be a quotation from one of Diocles' (lost) works. See van der Eijk, 2001: 79–82; Schöner, 1964: 72; Nutton, 2004: 123; 2005: 117–118. In addition, we find in a letter, possibly written by Diocles to a King Antigonus, that four different fluids in the body are said to increase at different times of the year. Frg. 183a (van der Eijk) = (Dubious), Paul of Aegina, Medical Excerpts, 1.100.1–6 (CMG IX 1, vol. 1, p. 68,25–72,12 Heiberg). The provenance of this letter is a complex issue, with a large number of versions of this letter produced with different attributions to both sender and recipient. This version by Paul of Aegina is considered by van der Eijk to be the closest to the original. However, the authenticity of this letter is still controversial. See van der Eijk, 2001: 352–358; Nutton, 2005: 117–118. See also Schöner, 1964: 73. There is also a passage in *Anonymus Parisinus*, about Diocles' theory that 'melancholy' (μελαγχολία) is caused when black bile gathers around the heart, which can affect a person's mental faculties. Frg. 108 (van der Eijk) = *Anonymus Parisinus, On Acute and Chronic Diseases* 19 (p. 116,22–118,2 Garofalo). See Flashar, 1966: 50–54; van der Eijk, 2001: 214–215. This seems to suggest, as van der Eijk points out, that Diocles can be regarded as basing his explanation of health and disease in the body on a humoral theory that has some significant similarities to the ideas contained in *On the Nature of Man*. However, the controversy surrounding the reliability of these sources, along with the lack of direct detail on Diocles' use of humoral theory, means that it is not possible to determine whether Diocles fully adopted the four-humour system of *On the Nature of Man*. Further to this, van der Eijk has questioned whether Galen can be fully trusted as a source for information on Diocles relating to the four humours. See van der Eijk, 2001: 48 and 86–87.

as blood, phlegm, yellow bile and black bile.[49] But, this type of theory cannot be associated with the four-humour system of *On the Nature of Man*. Most significantly, black bile does not play a major role in Plato's explanation of the causes of disease in relation to blood, phlegm and bile.[50] In a similar way, the med-

---

49 In the *Timaeus* we find that, for Plato, the most fundamental substances are the four cosmic elements; fire, water, air and earth. Plato, *Ti.* 32b; *Anon. Lond.* XIV,11–15 and 26–32; cf. Gal., *PHP*, VIII.2.21, CMG V 4,1,2, p. 494,22–25 De Lacy (V 667,3–6 K). Plato defines three separate categories for the cause of diseases in the body. The first type of causation is when the four elements, fire, air, water and earth are in excess, deficiency, or change into an unnatural state in relation to the proportion of the four qualities, hot, cold, dry and wet. The second category of causation of diseases occurs when there is a reversal of the natural process of nutrition in the body. In Plato's theory, the body is healthy when the homoeomerous parts of the body, such as the flesh and bone, are nourished by the blood, which provides the essential substances. However, diseases are produced when there is a breakdown of these parts into noxious substances, such as phlegm and bile, which are taken into the blood. Therefore, these two humours are residues from the decomposition of the homoeomerous parts of the body. The third type of disease is caused by pneuma, phlegm and bile. This is related to problems in the lungs when the pathways become blocked and restrict the movement of air to parts of the body. Black bile is mentioned briefly when it is said to cause problems when mixed with 'white phlegm'. It is referenced also in relation to a type of blood that is derived from black and acid bile, which in turn is associated with a substance in the body called 'acid phlegm'. Inflammations are said to be caused by the heat from bile, which involves the mixing of bile with blood, which displaces the natural fibrin in the blood. Plato, *Ti.* 81e–86a; *Anon. Lond.* XVII,11–XVIII,8. See Cornford, 1937: 334-340; Schöner, 1964: 63–64 and Lloyd, 2003: 154. Therefore, in Plato's medical theory, health and disease in the body are dependent on the blending of the four cosmic elements, fire, air, water and earth. The humours appear as a secondary explanation of disease, but these are generated as residues in the body when decomposition occurs. This is very different from the four-humour system found in the Hippocratic *On the Nature of Man*, but this has not prevented Galen from listing Plato as following Hippocrates' theory of the humours. Galen attempts to justify this claim further in *On the Doctrines of Hippocrates and Plato*, where he quotes from the *Timaeus* and argues that Plato actually intended to write about the four humours, which we find in *On the Nature of Man*. *PHP*, VIII.4.24–35, CMG V 4,1,2, pp. 504,3–506,3 De Lacy (V 677,6–679,16 K); cf. Plato, *Ti.* 82c and *Anon. Lond.* XV,20–36. If we look at the different categories of Plato's theory of diseases in the *Timaeus*, the first type based on the four cosmic elements is not a humoral theory. But the second and third types, which refer to phlegm and bile in different forms as humours, can be considered to be a type of humoral theory, similar to that of Philolaus.

50 Lloyd refers to the question of whether the material relating to humours as the cause of diseases in the *Timaeus* reflects Plato's view or whether it is actually the medical theory of someone else, with Philistion and Philolaus being named as possible sources. However, I agree with Lloyds' argument that the *Anonymus Londinensis* has clearly distinguished this theory as being by Plato and not that of Philistion and Philolaus. In addition, even if Plato is drawing heavily upon these types of sources, it is important to understand how he presents the material in his writing. See Lloyd, 2003: 153; cf. Cornford, 1937: 333–341. For example, Plato's concept of a cause of disease relating to a restriction of air to move in and

ical theories of Praxagoras, Pleistonicus and Phylotimus, indicate that there are different types of humoral theory being used. But these are not related to the four-humour system of *On the Nature of Man*. Instead, we find that the humours are regarded as types of waste products that can cause disease due to the effect of different types of qualities at certain places in the body. This is significant for black bile, as this substance is more generally characterised as a type of physiological or pathogenic residue in the medical texts, with the notable exception of *On the Nature of Man*.[51] Finally, humoral theory is not used in the writing of Aristotle and Theophrastus. Aristotle based his concept of the

---

out of the body is similar to Philistion's ideas concerning air in the body. However, Plato's theory is different, as he adds phlegm and bile to air as the cause of disease. See Nutton, 2004: 116–118. In Galen's opinion, Plato is the author of the medical writing in the *Timaeus*, as Galen quotes sections of this treatise in some of his works and attributes them to Plato.

51   There is clearer evidence for Galen's manipulation of the work of Praxagoras of Cos, and some of his students, in relation to the Hippocratic *On the Nature of Man*. Starting with Praxagoras himself, we find that he postulated ten different types of humour for his theory of health and disease in the body. He calls the humours of phlegm: sweet (γλυκύς), equally mixed (ἰσόκρατος) and vitreous (ὑαλοειδής). Other humours are named: acidic (ὀξύς), caustic (νιτρώδης), salty (ἁλυκός) and bitter (πικρός). Then there are the humours that are named due to their colour, such as leek-green (πρασοειδής) and yolk-coloured (λεκιθώδης). Finally, there is one humour that is called corrosive (ξυστικός). Galen considers blood as the eleventh humour of Praxagoras' theory: Frg. 21 (Steckerl) = Galen, *Nat. Fac.* II.9 (II 140,15–141,14 K). Cf. Frg. 22 (Steckerl) = Rufus of Ephesus, p. 165, 14 (Daremberg). See Nutton, 2005: 118. In *On the Natural Faculties*, Galen acknowledges the fact that Praxagoras has postulated ten humours, but explains it as an adoption of Hippocrates' system of four humours with a division into a range of species of humours to denote their different varieties. Galen, *Nat. Fac.* II.9 (II 141,4–8 K). This is an example of Galen's manipulation of material that is related to the humours, which he presents as being part of a systematic development of a theory of four humours that has continued after Hippocrates. Blood is not included among these ten humours, and Steckerl suggests that Galen has interpreted Praxagoras' ten humours as being a division of the phlegm, yellow bile and black bile of the four-humour system in the Hippocratic *On the Nature of Man*. But Steckerl argues that this interpretation by Galen may be a manipulation of Praxagoras' work and that Praxagoras may not have been aware of the Hippocratic four-humour system. See Steckerl, 1958: 9–10. There is a similar case for Phylotimus and Pleistonicus, two of Praxagoras' students. Both are thought to have adopted a similar humoral theory to their master, but Galen tells us that Phylotimus refers to a thick (παχύς), glutinous (κολλώδης) and cold (ψυχρός) humour that can be produced in the body by foodstuffs such as barley cake (μάζα). *Alim. Fac.* I.12, CMG V 4,2, p. 234,1–3 Helmreich (VI 509,14–16 K). In Phylotimus' *On Food*, there are many references to the humours of different qualities described by Praxagoras: *Athen. Deipnosoph.* II.53; II.81; III.79. See Steckerl, 1958: 108–113 and 124–126; De Lacy, 1980: 689–690; Nutton, 2005: 118. However, Galen is not justified in aligning the work of Praxagoras, Phylotimus and Pleistonicus with Hippocrates' humoral system and from the evidence that we possess, we do not find black bile (or the other three humours) being referred to explicitly in the theory of disease of these three physicians.

human body on four qualities; hot, cold, dry and wet.[52] When Aristotle refers to blood, phlegm, yellow bile and black bile, he does so as 'residues' (περιττώ-ματα), which are the waste products of bodily functions, such as the digestion of food.[53] Therefore, contrary to Galen's statement, Aristotle did not in any way follow the ideas contained in *On the Nature of Man* in his writing about the role of the humours in health and disease. In fact, Aristotle's theory of disease is not based on a humoral theory at all.[54] Galen's listing of Theophrastus as following Hippocrates' theory of humours is also unjustified, as the evidence suggests that Theophrastus adopted Aristotle's theory of the elements and qualities and so would probably have had a similar view about the function of black bile.[55] The reason that Galen attempts to collect together these earlier authorities and present them as if they are in agreement with a four-humour system of Hippocrates is to provide him with a powerful argument against his rivals, such as the Erasistrateans and the followers of Asclepiades.[56]

---

52 In *Generation and Corruption*, Aristotle pairs up the qualities into four compounds: hot and dry, hot and wet, cold and wet, and cold and dry. These four compounds are then associated with the four cosmic elements: fire, air, water and earth. So we then have fire being hot and dry, air is hot and wet, water is cold and wet and finally, earth is cold and dry. For Aristotle, fire and earth are the purest elements, whereas water and air are more mixed. Aristotle, *GC*, II.3, 330a30–b5 and 330b32–331a6. See Schöner, 1964: 66–67.

53 Aristotle, *HA*, III.2, 511b1–11. See van der Eijk, 2001: 48. When it comes to his characterisation of the individual humours, Aristotle describes blood as being hot and wet, and sweet in flavour and red in colour. It is associated with the heart, which is the principal location of heat in the body. Aristotle, *HA*, III.19, 520b10–33; *PA*, IV.2, 677a20–29. See Schöner, 1964: 68. Aristotle never explicitly uses the term 'four humours', as Galen does, and we do not find them being collectively used to explain health and disease in the body. Aristotle also refers to black bile as a type of moisture (ὑγρός), which can affect the sight of melancholic people. This black bile, being a cold substance, affects the heart and the area surrounding it, which is also the nutritive region in Aristotle's physiological theory. *HA*, III.2, 511b10–11; *Somn. Vig.* III, 457a32–34. See van der Eijk, 2005: 141–143.

54 As van der Eijk points out, the only place where phlegm, yellow bile and black bile are found together in a single passage is *On the History of Animals*, where these three humours are listed alongside faeces as residues. In addition, these humours are not referred to as residues (περιττώματα) in the extant Hippocratic Corpus. See van der Eijk, 2005: 153; cf. Schöner, 1964: 67.

55 Sharples, 1995: 10–16; 1998: 42–45; 56–58; 86–88; 113–116 and 119–121.

56 See Vegetti, 1999b: 387–395.

3   Summary

There are some important issues that relate to Galen's selection of the four-humour system from the Hippocratic *On the Nature of Man* as the best theory of how proximate elements can explain health and disease in the body. We have found that Galen is committed to the inclusion of black bile as a fundamental substance in the body, even though this is not the case for many other medical writers both within the Hippocratic Corpus, and outside of it, with the notable exception of the writer of *On the Nature of Man*. Galen goes further and associates this four-humour theory, not only with Hippocrates himself, but also with some of the most prominent physicians and philosophers of the fourth and third centuries BCE. In this way, Galen is attempting to support his claim for the superiority of the four humours, which is found to be mainly unsubstantiated from the evidence that we possess. However, on the contrary, it is clear that the four-humour system of *On the Nature of Man* is only one among a large number of humoral and non-humoral theories. Therefore, Galen creates a false status of black bile as one of the most important substances in ancient medicine. This shows part of Galen's strategy to manipulate the writing of some of the key authorities in the past to support his arguments against anyone who is critical of Hippocrates and denies the importance of black bile in the theory of the cause of health and disease in the body. When Galen does this, he suppresses important information about black bile in two ways. Firstly, there are some cases where black bile is characterised as a physiological or pathogenic residue. Secondly, we can find some treatises where black bile is not mentioned at all. This applies both to a large number of treatises in the Hippocratic Corpus, but also to the many different types of theory of disease that have been produced by philosophers and physicians over several centuries, from the fifth century BCE onwards. This leaves Galen with a problem of explaining how black bile can be responsible for diseases that have symptoms of pustules and that cause harm to bodily tissue, if he only uses the description of black bile found in *On the Nature of Man*. We shall see that Galen overcomes this potential problem by expanding the characterisation of black bile beyond the ideas contained in *On the Nature of Man*. He does this by utilising information on black bile from a number of sources, such as other texts from the Hippocratic Corpus, material from Plato and Aristotle, and some of the physicians that he has named as following Hippocrates' humoral system.

CHAPTER 2

Key Influences on Galen's Writing on Black Bile

In this chapter I will discuss the important issues relating to the most significant influences on Galen's writing about black bile. Firstly, I will summarise the
importance of philosophy on Galen's medical writing, particularly concerning
his ideas on elemental theory and teleology and how this also influenced his
view of the Hippocratic writings. I then move on to what is currently known
about the development of the medical texts attributed to Hippocrates, which
were collected at the library of Alexandria starting in the late fourth century
BCE.[1] There is some evidence to show that this collection of medical texts
was read, commented on, glossed and edited by some of the most prominent
physicians from the fourth century BCE up to the time of Galen in the second century CE. This is useful to provide a background on the general view
of the 'Hippocratic Corpus' when Galen started to train as a physician. This
will help us to understand how Galen approaches issues concerning the consistency of authorship of the different Hippocratic works. The main section of
this chapter contains analysis of Galen's view of the authenticity of some of
the texts from the Hippocratic Corpus on the basis of language and doctrine.
Here, I only refer to the Hippocratic texts that I have used for my research,
rather than including all the known treatises from the Hippocratic Corpus. My
selection of Hippocratic treatises is based on two main factors. Some texts are
chosen because they contain material on black bile or phenomena relating to
this humour. Others are selected because they are important for some points
of comparison with Galen's use of black bile in his medical writing, but do not
actually contain material on black bile. We shall see that Galen has manipu-
lated some of the ideas contained in the Hippocratic Corpus and the works of
these philosophers and physicians to make it seem that a four-humour system
has been used and developed by some of the important medical authorities in
the several centuries after the fifth century BCE. Galen uses this in his polemical arguments to refute the theories that explain health and disease in the
body that were used by his rivals, such as Erasistratus and Asclepiades. One
particular aim of this chapter is to explain the reasons why Galen has identified the first part of *On the Nature of Man* as being written by Hippocrates,

---

1 See Vallance, 2000: 95–113.

despite this treatise not being included in the list of best and most genuine Hippocratic works by earlier commentators.

1   The Importance of Philosophy in Galen's Interpretation of the Hippocratic Corpus

In the previous chapter we found that it was not just physicians of the past that Galen draws upon to support his assertion for humoral theory and in particular black bile. Philosophers, such as Plato and Aristotle, were also used as authorities and were portrayed as followers of Hippocratic humoral theory. Galen's view is that philosophy is the basis for understanding medicine, as he makes it clear that he considers Hippocrates to be the first physician who has demonstrated the correct philosophical methodology for medicine.[2] We find that Galen draws attention to philosophical methodology, such as the ability to distinguish between genus and species, and the importance of logical theory.[3] Galen is concerned with the general lack of commitment to intellectual study in society, as he believes that some physicians working in the second century CE not only neglect training in this type of methodology, but also are critical of people that undertake it.[4] For Galen, a doctor must not just acknowledge the importance of philosophy in medicine, but he must train hard in developing the skills from philosophy that are useful in medical practice. This is part of the ethical and serious attitude to knowledge that can only come through philosophy.[5] Galen ends this work with the advice that 'true followers of Hippocrates'

---

2   For example in *Opt. Med.* (1 (I 53,3–55,7 K)), Galen describes Hippocrates as an ideal physician who should be emulated. See Smith, 1979: 83–96 and Mattern, 2008: 8–9.

3   Here Galen refers to genus (γένος) and species (εἶδος), which we also find in Aristotelian biological taxonomy. In this system genus is a grouping according a unique feature, such as wings, which are not shared by other groups. The species relates to the different forms within a genus group, such as birds have wings, or fish have fins. This can also be applied to different levels of generality. See Balme, 1987: 72.

4   Galen argues that a doctor must know all the parts of philosophy, which he defines as 'the logical, the physical and the ethical' (τό τε λογικὸν, καὶ τό φυσικὸν, καὶ τό ἠθικόν). The inclusion of ethics applies to the doctor's conduct in practising medicine, which should move him towards a more temperate lifestyle (σωφροσύνη). Gal. *Opt. Med.* 1 and 3 (I 53,1–55,9 and 60,10–61,8 K). The division of philosophy into the three categories: logic, physics and ethics can also be found in Stoicism, but Galen is not advocating this philosophical school as the one to follow, or indeed any particular philosophical school. See Aëtius, I, Preface 2 (LS 26A); Diogenes Laertius, 7.39–41 (LS 26B); Plutarch, *On Stoic self-contradictions*, 1035A (LS 26C).

5   Hankinson, 2008: 210–211; Chiaradonna, 2014: 61 and Singer 2014: 9.

('Ιπποκράτους ἀληθῶς ... ζηλωταί) should consider philosophy as 'foremost' (πρό-τερον), giving the overall impression of Hippocrates' superior ability in philoso-phy and his deployment of it within the field of medicine.[6] We can understand why Galen would highlight ethics as being important in Hippocrates' writing, as he could point to examples of what he considered the best practice for physi-cians in the Hippocratic Corpus.

For Galen, the importance of logic in medicine was the ability to discover the truth. So we find in *On the Therapeutic Method*, Galen's claim that logic can discern truth from falsehood. Here, Galen is referring to a methodology of logic, which can produce a demonstration. This is constructed from premises (accepted as being true) and by a process of deduction to provide a conclu-sion. This method, which Galen classifies as 'demonstrative' (ἀποδεικτική), is the standard for what he considers as proof that something is true.[7] This term is used by Galen many times to say that Hippocrates has proven something. For example, in *On the Elements According to Hippocrates*, Galen tells us that Hip-pocrates has proven that the fundamental element in the body cannot be one in form and power and that the four qualities are the elements of all things in the universe.[8] Galen emphasises Hippocrates' use of the demonstrative method, as he claims that Hippocrates developed a method that can determine the 'nature' of the elements, such as knowing if they are just one, or many, and identifying their particular characteristics. However, as Leith points out, a fully developed methodology of this type does not appear in *On the Nature of Man*, but it can be found in Aristotle's *Physics*.[9] In this way Galen is manipulating the ideas con-tained in *On the Nature of Man* in order to create a 'history' of the development of this methodology to examine natural phenomena, which has Hippocrates as the founder, and then a later development by authorities such as Aristotle. We saw a similar strategy when Galen listed the physicians and philosophers that have followed Hippocrates' four-humour theory.[10]

One important area of philosophy is teleology, which Galen uses in his bio-logical theory. When it comes to his writing on black bile, Galen's use of teleol-

---

6   *Opt. Med.* 4 (I 62,16–63,4 K).

7   *MM*, I.2.2 (X 8,17–9,12 and 18 K); *Ord. Lib. Prop.* 1 (XIX 50,5–8 K). See Morison, 2008: 68–69.

8   Gal. *Hipp. Elem.* 2.8; 10.1, CMG V 1,2, pp. 58,22–26; 138,15–18 De Lacy (I 416,9–13; 492,3–7 K); cf. *Nat. Fac.* I.2 (II 5,8–13 K). There are many other examples of Galen using the term ἀπόδειξις to report that Hippocrates has proven something important in medicine.

9   Gal. *Hipp. Elem.* 2.1–2, CMG V 1,2, p. 58,6–10 De Lacy (I 415,4–10 K); Aristotle, *Ph.* 1.2, 184b15–22. See Leith, 2014: 215–216; Hankinson, 2009: 233.

10 See chapter 1, section 2 above.

ogy is important in two ways. Firstly, in *On the Natural Faculties*, Galen defends
the very existence of black bile on the basis of teleology. Secondly, in *On the
Utility of the Parts*, Galen uses teleology to explain the spleen's purpose to reg-
ulate and remove black bile from the body. This second point is part of Galen's
overall view of causation in the body, which he uses to attack the theories of
the Atomists and physicians, such as Asclepiades. For example, in *On the Natural Faculties*, Galen puts forward his own case for teleology as the most likely
cause for the explanation of the nature of the most fundamental phenomena
in the universe.[11] In another example from *On the Utility of the Parts*, Galen
claims that Aristotle's teleological system is superior to Plato's for the explanation of anatomy and physiology. However, neither Aristotle nor Plato have
been able to combine teleology within a biological theory to explain how the
parts of body are formed in the way they are and how they function. At this
point, Galen even admits that Hippocrates was not able to achieve this.[12] This
brings us to a particular issue in Galen's presentation of the history of the development of teleological models that he uses to present his own ideas. When it
comes to the originator of the role of a purposeful and intelligent agent at work
in the universe, it is not Plato or Aristotle that Galen names as the first person
to develop this type of theory, but Hippocrates. Instead, the work of Plato and
Aristotle on teleology is acknowledged by Galen as following on from the original ideas of Hippocrates.[13] Galen's emphasis on Hippocrates as the foremost
teleologist is, as Flemming points out, fraudulent when it comes to the actual
content of the Hippocratic Corpus. This was part of Galen's reinforcement of
his own work to be in agreement with the work of Hippocrates and since he
wants to refute the materialistic theories with arguments about teleology, then
he requires there to be a Hippocratic basis for them, with Platonic and Aristotelian teleology being secondary to the work of Hippocrates.[14] In order to
achieve a Hippocratic origin for teleology in medicine, Galen gives examples
of the instances where Hippocrates has referred to Nature as being creative
and active in designing living beings. For example in *On the Natural Faculties*,
we have: 'Nature acts skilfully and decently throughout' (ἡ φύσις ἅπαντα τεχνι-
κῶς καὶ δικαίως πράττει), which Galen attributes to Hippocrates' writing. In *On
the Utility of the Parts*, Galen says that Hippocrates is 'continually singing the
praises of Nature's righteousness and the foresight she displays in the creation

---

11   For example, *Nat. Fac.* I,7 (II 26,14–27,16 K). See Lloyd, 1996: 266–267; Gill, 2010: 66–67.
12   Flemming, 2009: 66–67.
13   Smith, 1979: 86.
14   Flemming, 2009: 72.

of animals' (διὰ παντὸς ὑμνοῦντι τὴν δικαιοσύνην αὐτῆς καὶ τὴν εἰς τὰ ζῷα πρόνοιαν) and attributes to Hippocrates, the following: 'Nature is well-trained, just, skilful, and provident in her treatment of animals' (ὡς εὐπαίδευτός τε καὶ δικαία καὶ τεχνικὴ καὶ προνοητικὴ τῶν ζῴων ἡ φύσις ἐστίν).[15] However, there is a problem, as we do not find these terms being applied to 'Nature' in the Hippocratic Corpus in the way that Galen claims that they are. For example, in the case of 'well-trained' (εὐπαίδευτος), the author of the Hippocratic *On Joints* uses this term to describe surgery attendants, rather than a providential Nature.[16] In addition to this, Galen also brings in various passages and remarks from Hippocratic texts out of context in order to strengthen his case for Hippocratic teleology. In *On the Doctrines of Hippocrates and Plato*, Galen quotes the following three Hippocratic passages: 'Nature, being well-instructed, does what is needed without being taught' (εὐπαίδευτος ἡ φύσις ἐοῦσα, οὐ μαθοῦσα τὰ δέοντα ποιέει), 'Our natures are the physicians of our diseases' (φύσιες νούσων οἱ ἰητροί) and 'Nature will wholly suffice' (φύσις ἐξαρκέσει παντάπασι). He uses these passages as examples of Hippocrates' admiration for the power of Nature, naming it as the cause that fashioned human beings.[17] The first two statements come from the fifth section of *Epidemics VI* and the third one is from *On Nutriment*. As Flemming suggests, these phrases do not conflict with Galen's view of 'Nature' (φύσις), but they do not provide enough information to justify his argument for a fully developed Hippocratic teleology that is the basis of the later work by Plato and Aristotle.[18] This is the way that Galen manipulates Hippocratic texts and draws upon different passages from different works, as if they are presented as offering a coherent argument in the way that Galen requires.[19] Galen attempts to make a case for a Hippocratic precedent for purposiveness in Nature, when he uses the notion that 'Nature is Just' (δικαία ἡ φύσις) in *On the Utility of the Parts*.[20]

---

15 *Nat. Fac.* I.12 (II 30 K); *UP*, III.10; V.9 (III 235,6–8; 379,10–11 K), translations by May. See Flemming, 2009: 73.

16 *Artic.* XLIII (IV 186,5–8 L). See May, 1968: 264, note 33. In *Epidemics VI* there is another instance of 'well-trained' being applied in a context that is closer to Galen's notion of 'Nature', see below.

17 *PHP*, IX.8.26–27, CMG V 4,1,2, p. 596,21–29 De Lacy (V 790,16–791,8 K). See Flemming, 2009: 73.

18 *Epid. VI*, V (V 314,5–8 L); *Alim.*, XV (IX 102,16 L); Flemming, 2009: 73. Galen does acknowledge the Hippocratic content of *Epidemics VI* and regards *On Nutriment* as an example of a genuine work by Hippocrates, see Craik, 2015: 23 and 89.

19 Jouanna suggests that Galen is using the connection between two adjectives: 'untaught' (ἀδίδακτος) and 'uneducated' (ἀπαιδεύτος) and the substitution of the singular φύσις for its plural in order to make the combination of these two sources more convincing. See Jouanna, 2002b: 253–254.

20 For example: *UP*, I.22; II.16 (III 81,10; 158,6–9 K). See Flemming, 2009: 73.

In this case, we do find the use of δικαία and φύσις together in the Hippocratic *On Fractures* and *On Joints*. However, again, as Flemming points out, the Hippocratic context is more to do with the setting of bone or a dislocation in a way that most conforms to what is most natural.[21] Therefore, this may be a deliberate manipulation of the Hippocratic Corpus to support Galen's assertion for a clear teleological basis of Hippocrates' writing on physiology and anatomy, which Galen can use alongside the more explicitly defined teleological material in the works of Plato and Aristotle.

2   The Influence of Galen's Teachers on His Views Concerning Medical Theory

In addition to philosophy, we must investigate the influence of Galen's teachers for an understanding of his writing on black bile. Galen was writing in the period of the so-called 'Second Sophistic', which von Staden characterises as an epideictic culture that favoured public displays, re-enactment of Greek historical events, particularly from the fifth and fourth century BCE, along with an interest in the Attic language.[22] Therefore, Galen's use of material from the Greek classical period of the fifth and fourth century BCE to support his arguments and theories can be viewed within this context.[23] One particular debate that Galen took an active interest in was the 'Hippocratic Question', which is based on the issues of how to reliably decide the authenticity of the large amount of texts that make up the Hippocratic Corpus. We find throughout Galen's writing many references and quotes to passages that he labels as being by Hippocrates or that are in agreement with Hippocratic doctrine. In order to understand how Galen made decisions about material from treatises, I want to try to determine what the 'Hippocratic Corpus' actually was in the second century CE because Galen did not analyse treatises from the Hippocratic Corpus without reference to earlier studies on these texts. The various treatises that comprise the Hippocratic Corpus were originally used and collected together from the fourth century BCE onwards. The reason why so many medical texts were brought together during this period was a move towards a

---

21   *Fract.* I; XXXVII (III 412,3–414,1; 540,16–17 L); *Artic.* XLVII; LXII; LXX (IV 210,1–4; 266,13–17; 288,12–14 L). See Flemming, 2009: 73. See also Jouanna's analysis of Galen's manipulation of the Hippocratic works to present his argument that Hippocrates already had developed the concept of teleology from his use of a 'just Nature': Jouanna, 2002b: 252.
22   Von Staden, 1997a: 33.
23   Harig and Kollesch 1975: 270–271; Swain, 1996: 378.

more systematic development of medicine, which required a consistent rational approach to the causes of health and disease. This process began with a number of physicians choosing to develop their medical theories in this rationalistic way. However, at this early point in the history of medicine, there did not seem to be any acknowledgement of Hippocrates or Hippocratic medicine as the best authority and foundation of this new rationalist thinking.[24] We can obtain an understanding of the Hippocratic writings from the way that they were used by physicians and those interested in medical texts. For example, it was thought that the physician Diocles of Carystus (fourth century BCE) was a good, early source for the interpretation of Hippocratic doctrine. However, this is now not considered to be the case and analysis conducted by scholars, such as Smith and van der Eijk, have cast doubt on the usefulness of Diocles to analyse the early view of the Hippocratic works.[25] Therefore, we need to look elsewhere to investigate the early collection of medical texts that were designated as being by 'Hippocrates'.

In the early Hellenistic period, the library at Alexandria had collected a large amount of medical works, many of which became attributed to Hippocrates.[26] One of the most prominent physicians at this time was Herophilus (325–250 BCE), who was well regarded because of his pioneering work on anatomy and physiology from his studies on human dissection and vivisection. Earlier we saw that the evidence indicates that Herophilus probably did not follow Hippocrates' humoral system in the way that Galen has suggested.[27] However, it

---

24   Lloyd discusses the problems involved in attempting to provide a modern solution to the 'Hippocratic Question'. His conclusion is that it is clear that what we call the Hippocratic Corpus is actually a collection of texts by a large number of different writers. Information on Hippocrates from ancient sources, such as Plato, Aristotle, Hellenistic writers and Galen, do not provide reliable enough evidence for us to make a conclusive determination of the Hippocratic authenticity of any of the treatises. See Lloyd, 1975; Smith, 1979: 177–178.

25   Smith argues that if Diocles had said anything significant about Hippocrates, whether it was in praise or to criticise him, then it would be highly likely that Galen would have reported this somewhere in the texts that have survived. But this does not mean that Diocles was unaware of Hippocrates and it is likely that he did read some of these works, such as *On Regimen*. It has been suggested by van der Eijk that the evidence to associate Diocles with Hippocratic medicine is inconclusive. But, he does concede that it is possible for Diocles to have been aware of at least some of the Hippocratic works. See Smith, 1979: 187 and 189–191; van der Eijk, 2001: xxxiii and xxxv; von Staden, 2006a: 16.

26   *Hipp. Epid.* III.II.4, CMG V 10,2,1, pp. 78,27–80,6 Wenkebach (XVIIa 605,10–608,1 K). See Smith, 1979: 199–202; Small, 1997: 44; Vallance, 2000: 95–101.

27   See chapter 1, section 2 above.

is likely that Herophilus engaged with the Hippocratic works, but it is doubtful that he wrote commentaries on any of them.[28] What we find is that there was a more active engagement with the collection of Hippocratic texts among his followers. For example, the Herophilean Bacchius of Tanagra (c. 275–200 BCE) wrote commentaries on *Aphorisms*, *Epidemics VI* and *In the Surgery*.[29] Then there are the Empiricists, a rival group to the Herophileans, who are also important for this early work on the Hippocratic texts. The evidence in the extant sources indicates that the Empiricist Zeuxis (most likely c. 250–175 BCE) worked on six Hippocratic texts: *On Places in Man*, *Aphorisms*, *Prorrhetic I*, *Epidemics II*, *III* and *VI*.[30] Another Empiricist, Glaucias of Tarentum, who was a contempo-

---

28 Von Staden suggests that although Herophilus offered critical responses to a few of the Hippocratic texts, such as *Prognostic*, and glossed some Hippocratic words and expressions, the precise literary form that he used is not clear. Von Staden cites Caelius Aurelianus (T31 and T261, *Tardae passiones*, 4.8.113) and Gal. (T32 and T264, *Hipp. Prog.* 1.4, CMG V 9,2, p. 204,4–205,8 Heeg (XVIIIb 13,14–16,4 K)) for evidence of Herophilus' writing against the Hippocratic *Prognostic*. But, this does not necessarily imply that Herophilus had written a commentary on the *Prognostic*. See Smith, 1979: 191–193 and 199; von Staden, 1982: 78 and 90; 1989: 74–76; 2006a: 16; Hanson, 1998: 37; Vallance, 2000, 101 and 107.

29 Von Staden claims that the modern view that Bacchius wrote commentaries on *On the Nature of the Child*, *Epidemics II* and *III* is based on inconclusive evidence. See von Staden, 2006a: 17–18 and 20–25. See also Hanson, 1998: 37–38; Vallance, 2000: 102. In the case of *In the Surgery*, Galen includes Bacchius among the earliest commentators of this text. He found this version useful, not only for its 'ancient readings', but also for the inclusion of some variants of its reading that were in agreement among the very earliest commentators on this text. However, in contrast to this praise, we find that Galen accused Bacchius, among other early commentators, of making emendations to the transmitted text of *Epidemics VI*. Bacchius also wrote a glossary on Hippocratic works, not only to explain obscure and difficult medical terms, but also to show where common language was used in a medical context. *Hipp. Off. Med.* Pref. (XVIIIb 631,9–632,1 K); *Hipp. Epid.* (VI) Pref. CMG V 10,2,2, pp. 3,4–4,6 Wenkebach (XVIIa 793,4–794,10 K); *Hipp. Epid.* III.II.25, CMG V 10,2,1, pp. 87,6–15 Wenkebach (XVIIa 618,19–619,11 K). See Smith, 1979: 202–204; von Staden, 1999a: 158; 2006a: 18–20 and 26–27.

30 Galen reports that Zeuxis wrote commentaries on 'all books of Hippocrates', but as von Staden points out, it is unclear whether this means the texts that Galen believes are authentic or all the books attributed to Hippocrates at that time. If it is the former, then this would be one of the first attempts at a comprehensive exegesis of a Hippocratic Corpus. Galen reports Zeuxis' gloss of the Hippocratic *On Places in Man* in his *Gloss.* (XIX 107,14–108,5 K). The evidence for Zeuxis' commentary on *Prorrhetic I* comes from a passage in Galen's own commentary on this Hippocratic work (*Hipp. Prorrh.* II.23, CMG V 9,2, p. 73,8–20 Diels (XVI 636,5–637,4 K)). There is a reference to Zeuxis' interpretation of the Hippocratic *Aphorisms* when Galen is discussing the analysis of a particular aphorism by the early authorities. Von Staden suggests that this indicates a commentary on *Aphorisms* by Zeuxis, as Galen is referring to a set of early commentators, who go further than lexicography and glossary of terms (*Hipp. Aph.* VII.69 (XVIIIa

rary of Zeuxis, provided interpretation of some passages from *Epidemics VI*.[31] Unfortunately, information on the work of these early Hellenistic Herophileans and Empiricists only survives in fragments or in remarks made by later writers, such as Erotian, Celsus and Galen.[32]

In addition to the Herophileans and Empiricists, there are other physicians who engaged with the Hippocratic works. In his *Commentary on In the Surgery*, Galen includes Asclepiades, alongside Bacchius, Zeuxis and Heraclides of Tarentum, in his list of early Hippocratic commentators.[33] Asclepiades of Bithynia (second to first century BCE) had a reputation of opposing 'Hippocratic' medicine, which is a view that Galen has encouraged in his polemical arguments against him. It was thought that Asclepiades had written two commentaries, one on the Hippocratic *In the Surgery* and the other on *Aphorisms*. However, new evidence suggests that he also wrote a commentary on the Hip-

---

186,11–187,4 κ)). The evidence for Zeuxis' commentary on *Epidemics II* is from just one source, which is a ninth century Arabic translation of Galen's commentary on this Hippocratic work (*Hipp. Epid.* II, CMG V 10,1 pp. 230,10–234,7 Pfaff). See von Staden, 2006a: 30–39.

31   For example, Galen criticised Glaucias for emending a passage from *Epidemics VI* in relation to information about the spleen (*Hipp. Epid.* VI, CMG V 10,2,2, pp. 451,40–452,2 Pfaff). See von Staden, 2006a: 40–44. There has been some generalisation that characterises the Empiricist interpretation of the Hippocratic texts solely on the basis of their empiricism, which was used to align 'Hippocrates' with their doctrine. This is the type of Empiricist strategy that was promoted by Galen in his polemic against some of the Empiricist physicians. However, analysis by von Staden suggests that some of the Empiricists adopted a more independent approach to their interpretation of the Hippocratic texts and in some cases defended a particular Herophilean view. For example, when Zeuxis comments on a passage from *Epidemics VI*, he attempts to defend the passage with reference to Herophilus' interpretation and even defends this view from the criticism of Herophileans, such as Callimachus. Further to this we find Zeuxis criticising Glaucias for tampering with the transmitted text of *Epidemics VI. Hipp. Epid.* VI.1.5; VI.11.43, CMG V 10,2,2, pp. 20,19–21,9; 114,1–9 Wenkebach (XVIIa 826,4–827,7; 992,9–16 κ). See von Staden, 2006a: 32–34 and 44–45. For an example of the view, which Galen promotes, that characterises Empiricist exegesis by associating empiricism with 'Hippocrates', see Smith, 1979: 177–178; 205; 208–210.

32   The earliest known, most 'complete', Hippocratic commentary is by the first century BCE Alexandrian physician, Apollonius of Citium. Smith reports that Apollonius, although sometimes writing in an Empiric style, did not refer to himself as an Empiricist. He is mostly positive about Hippocrates and the work that survives in his treatise *On Joints* draws heavily on the Hippocratic work of the same title. See Smith, 1979: 212–214; Nutton, 2004: 145.

33   Heraclides of Tarentum was an Empiricist from the first century BCE. He was a student of the Herophilean, Mantias. See von Staden, 1989: 86–87 and 106; Nutton, 2004: 144 and 151–152.

pocratic *Epidemics I*.[34] Galen was keen to characterise Asclepiades as being opposed to Hippocrates and there is evidence of Asclepiades criticising some parts of the Hippocratic texts, such as rejecting the theory of critical days. However, as Leith suggests, it is better to view Asclepiades' attitude towards Hippocrates as attempting to understand and provide a clear interpretation of the Hippocratic works, rather than trying to show that Hippocrates was at all times correct.[35] In this way, Asclepiades is closer to Herophilus' approach to Hippocrates. Another source on the work of Hippocrates comes from Celsus (first century CE), who attempted to create a 'history of medicine', which identifies Hippocrates as the first person to separate medicine from philosophy. Celsus constructs his historical narrative by emphasising Hippocrates' philosophical pedigree and by pointing out that he is sometimes called a student of Democritus and should be regarded as the founder of 'rationalist' medicine. We find that Celsus draws upon a wide range of Hippocratic works, but he does not attempt to ascertain the authenticity of the different texts that were attributed to Hippocrates.[36]

So far the information that we have on this early period of engagement with the texts that were collectively attributed to 'Hippocrates' is that the content was interpreted using glossaries, commentaries and edited versions of the treatises. However, we do not find evidence that there was a systematic study of the consistency of language and doctrine to determine the authenticity of individual or groups of texts. The first time we encounter a direct engagement with the question of the authenticity of Hippocratic works is in the first century CE. It is at this time that Erotian produced a 'Hippocratic' dictionary to help his fellow physicians to access the large amount of Hippocratic works available. Erotian accepts the authenticity of almost all the treatises, but he singles out *Prorrhetic II* as not being written by Hippocrates. However, we do

---

34   Galen's reference to Asclepiades as a commentator on the Hippocratic *In the Surgery* comes from *Hipp. Off. Med.* (Pref. (XVIIIb 631,9–632,1 K)). The evidence of Asclepiades' commentary on *Aphorisms* is from Caelius Aurelianus (*On Acute Diseases*, 3.1.3 (CML VI.1 p. 294 Bendz)) and *Epidemics I* is from a recently discovered papyrus (P. Oxy. LXXX 5231). See Leith, (forthcoming): 1–7. There has been some debate on whether Galen had access to only one of the texts from the four early commentators that he refers to in his *Commentary on In the Surgery*. Smith claims Asclepiades' commentary is the most likely one that Galen is using as his source. However, Leith has argued, on the basis of chronology, that if Galen only had one of these commentaries, it would most likely be by Heraclides. *Hipp. Off. Med.* I.5; I.22; II.29; II.30 (XVIIIb 666,10–14; 715,9–18; 805,16–806,2; 810,15–811,2 K). See Smith, 1979: 222–226; Leith, (forthcoming): 4.

35   Leith, (forthcoming): 15.

36   Celsus, *On Medicine*, pref. 7–10, 14–15, 47 and 66. See Smith, 1979: 226–230; von Staden, 1999b: 264–267; Nutton, 2004: 116.

not know why he rejected the authenticity of this particular text. For example, he might have been concerned about this treatise on the basis of linguistic or doctrinal issues.[37] Therefore, from the first century CE, we start to find more information on a debate within ancient medicine relating to the 'Hippocratic Question'. There is evidence that shows that physicians and medical commentators at this time became interested in comparing the Hippocratic treatises on the consistency of grammatical style and doctrinal content. This allowed them to determine whether a particular text was a genuine Hippocratic work or not. The first attested systematic investigation based on consistent criteria for the engagement with this 'Hippocratic Question' began with Dioscurides and Artemidorus Capiton at the beginning of the second century CE.[38] For example, we find that Dioscurides considered *On Diseases II* to be written by a person called Hippocrates, who was in fact the grandson of the more famous Hippocrates. He also believed that a certain passage from *Epidemics VI* was actually by Thessalos, rather than Hippocrates.[39] Galen tells us that Dioscurides had created a list of the treatises that he considered to be the 'most genuine and most useful works'. According to Galen, Dioscurides included *Aphorisms, Prognostic, On Regimen in Acute Diseases, Airs, Waters and Places*, and *Epidemics I* and *III* among the most genuine Hippocratic treatises.[40] It was the work of Dioscurides, and then Artemidorus after him, which brought together a set of texts, which could be collectively known as the Hippocratic Corpus.[41] The physician Rufus of Ephesus (first century CE) is another example of someone who actively engaged with the Hippocratic writings at this time. He wrote some commentaries on the Hippocratic texts, but these have unfortunately not survived.[42] Rufus was one of many physicians that attributed *On Diseases I* to Hippocrates, in contrast to Galen, who rejected it as inauthentic (see pages 49–50

---

37   It is possible that the question of Hippocratic authenticity may have been studied earlier than this. Smith considers the possibility that the earlier sources that Erotian was drawing on for his opinion may have left *Prorrhetic II* out of their glossaries for some reason. See Smith, 1979: 234; van der Eijk, 1999: 17; von Staden, 1999a: 187; Nutton, 2004: 212–213.

38   Smith, 1979: 234–236; Nutton, 2004: 213.

39   For Galen's presentation of Dioscurides' opinion on the authenticity of *Diseases II*, see *Hipp. Epid.* VI.I.29, CMG V 10,2,2, p. 55,16–56,10 Wenkebach (XVIIa 888,9–889,6 K); *HNH*, II.1, CMG V 9,1, p. 58,7–15 Mewaldt (XV 110,12–111,4 K). See Smith, 1979: 237; Roselli, 1999: 370.

40   *Hipp. Epid.* (III) Pref. CMG V 10,2,1, p. 60,4–61,13 Wenkebach (XVIIa 576,4–578,7 K). This was probably not an exhaustive list, but it does show that Dioscurides recognised a specific set of Hippocratic works as genuine. See Smith, 1979: 238–239.

41   Smith, 1979: 239–240; Nutton, 2004: 213.

42   Smith, 1979: 240–241; Pormann, 2008: 4–5; 135–136 and 146–149.

below).[43] Smith suggests that it seems likely that Galen used Rufus' commentaries as a source for his own writing on the Hippocratic works and that he read parts of Rufus' writing, which he found in the commentaries by Sabinus.[44]

This brings us to the period that just preceded Galen, with the main physicians working with Hippocratic texts being Marinus, his student Quintus, who in turn taught Lycus and Sabinus. Marinus is an important person in relation to Galen's view of the anatomical content of the Hippocratic Corpus. Galen respected Marinus' views on anatomy and, as Smith points out, he regards Marinus as the first to claim that *Epidemics II* contains information on the anatomy of the veins and nerves. Galen is critical of the rest of the content on anatomy in the Hippocratic writings as he believes that it is incorrect. Therefore, this one reference to a correct description of anatomy is essential for Galen to show that Hippocrates understood everything about the physiology and anatomy of the body.[45] When it comes to Quintus, Galen reports that he had not produced any published writing, but Galen uses him for some passages from the *Epidemics*, which Smith suggests may have come to Galen from his teacher Satyrus.[46] Galen was particularly hostile to Lycus, whom he criticises for failing to understand his own teacher (Quintus) and taking an Empiric stance when interpreting the Hippocratic works.[47] Sabinus published Hippocratic commentaries and was well regarded in the second century CE. He was a self-styled Hippocratean, and although Galen recommended some of his books, he was regarded by Galen as a rival in the competitive world of Roman society.[48]

---

43   Pormann, 2008: 148.

44   Smith, 1979: 243.

45   *Hipp. Epid.* II, CMG V 10,1, pp. 312,20–313,36; 330,39–331,8 Pfaff. See Smith, 1979: 65. Galen tells us that Marinus wrote some commentaries on Hippocratic works, but Smith is concerned that Galen does not mention these commentaries anywhere else in his extant writing. *Hipp. Epid.* VI, CMG V 10,2,2, pp. 286,27–288,36 Pfaff. In this commentary on *Epidemics VI*, Galen is quoting some of Lycus' reading of *Epidemics VI* and finds that it is based on the work of Marinus. Galen reports that there are many books attributed to Marinus in Rome, but he cannot find the one that refers to the relevant passage in *Epidemics VI*. See Smith, 1979: 65–68; Nutton, 2004: 219.

46   *Hipp. Epid.* VI, CMG V 10,2,2, pp. 314,18–20; 500, 38–39 Pfaff; II, CMG V 10,1, p. 222,41–42 Pfaff; *Ant.*, I.14 (XIV 69,5–12 K). See Smith, 1979: 68.

47   *Hipp. Epid.* III.I.4, CMG V 10,2,1, p. 14,12–17 Wenkebach (XVIIa 502,12–503,1 K). See Smith, 1979: 67–68.

48   *Hipp. Epid.* III.I.4, CMG V 10,2,1, p. 17,22–26 Wenkebach (XVIIa 507,18–508,5 K); II, CMG V 10,1, pp. 329,40–330,5 Pfaff. On one occasion, Galen defends some of Sabinus' commentary on *Aphorisms* against the view of Julian (one of Galen's own teachers): *Adv. Jul.* 3, CMG V 10,3, pp. 39,12–40,9 Wenkebach (XVIIIa 255,1–14 K). See Smith, 1979: 71–72; Nutton, 2004: 212.

We find that Sabinus is part of the general debate on the authenticity of *On the Nature of Man*, where Galen outlines his own view against that of Sabinus.

It is at this point that we reach a direct Hippocratic influence on Galen's early medical studies through some of his teachers. Galen had many teachers during his medical training, but there are four that are particularly important for Galen's writing on black bile because of their views on the Hippocratic writings. These are Numisianus and Satyrus, who were students of Quintus, and also Stratonicus (a student of Sabinus) and Pelops (a student of Numisianus).[49] Satyrus, a student of Quintus, wrote some Hippocratic commentaries, which may have been used by Galen when he wrote about his views of Quintus. We find that Galen references Satyrus in his *Commentary on Prorrhetic I*, as part of his general aim to refute the authenticity of this work (see pages 42–43 below).[50] Then there is Stratonicus, a student of Sabinus, who influenced Galen on Hippocratic medical practice, but like Quintus, did not publish anything. Galen quotes what he remembers from a lesson by Stratonicus, who interpreted a passage from *Epidemics VI* on the association between black bile and haemorrhoids. Galen believes that Stratonicus was following a traditional interpretation of this passage on black bile being normalised by haemorrhoids.[51] Pelops was very influential on Galen's medical training with reference to the Hippocratic works. He taught Galen about humoral pathology and even wrote a work called *Introduction to Hippocrates* along with many private commentaries on Hippocratic works, which Galen used in some of his own commentaries.[52] From these teachers, Galen gained training in medicine that used different

---

49 See Mattern, 2013: 36–80. Galen considered his teacher Numisianus, who was also a student of Marinus, to be superior in anatomy, but he complained that some parts of Numisianus' analysis of the Hippocratic works were inadequate. *AA*, I (II 217,17–218,4 K). There is also one passage from Galen's *Commentary on Epidemics II*, which tells us about Numisianus through Pelops, who was one of his students (and also a teacher of Galen). We are informed that Galen finds them both in error about the ability to infer temperament from external features (*Hipp. Epid.* II, CMG V 10,1, pp. 345,20–351,17 Pfaff). See Smith, 1979: 69; Mattern, 2013: 56–57.

50 *Hipp. Epid.* VI, CMG V 10,2,2, p. 412,30–413,1 Pfaff; *Hipp. Prorrh.* I.5, CMG V 9,2, p. 20,11–15 Diels (XVI 524,11–15 K). See Smith, 1979: 70; Mattern, 2013: 39–42 and 47–48.

51 *Hipp. Epid.* VI, CMG V 10,2,2, p. 303,12–16 and 412,24–26 Pfaff. See Smith, 1979: 70–71 and 132–133; Nutton, 2004: 212; Mattern, 2013: 58.

52 *Hipp. Epid.* VI, CMG V 10,2,2, p. 291,3–12 Pfaff. For Pelops' humoral pathology: *At. Bil.* 3.6, CMG V 4,1,1, p. 75,16–21 De Boer (V 112,13–113,1 K); *Hipp. Epid.* VI, CMG V 10,2,2, p. 500,14–21 Pfaff. For Pelops' commentaries: *Hipp. Epid.* VI, CMG V 10,2,2, pp. 412,31–413,1 Pfaff. For Pelops' 'Introduction to Hippocrates': *Musc. Diss.* XVIIIb 927,7–9 K. See Smith, 1979: 69–70; Nutton, 2004: 217; Mattern, 2013: 58.

methods to draw upon even the most obscure and brief passages in the Hippocratic writings. Galen then went on to develop his own style of 'reading' the Hippocratic treatises and using them to defend specific points in medical debates.[53]

3   Galen's Opinion on the Authenticity of the Hippocratic Writings

All of this shows that when Galen started to study medicine there was already a long tradition of interpretation and commentary on the texts of the Hippocrates writings. However, we have seen that there already had been some analysis on the consistency of language and doctrine of the different Hippocratic texts to ascertain authenticity. We know from his writing that Galen had access to the lists of 'authentic' Hippocratic works, such as the one compiled by Dioscurides, and he had also been taught by physicians who had their own opinion of what should be considered as genuine Hippocratic treatises. However, Galen did not just accept these views on Hippocratic authenticity without some analysis of his own. He wrote a specific book on his assessment of the authenticity of Hippocratic works, called *The Authentic and Spurious Writings of Hippocrates*, which demonstrates that he was actively involved with addressing this question on what constitutes a genuine Hippocratic text.[54] Unfortunately this text is now lost, but Galen does quote a small section from it in his *Commentary on On the Nature of Man*, which provides a short description of his method and criteria for the determination of genuine Hippocratic works:

> It contains a first account, where it expounds concerning the elements and humours, in accordance with the method of Hippocrates, as well as a second account, where it expounds on the differences between epidemic and sporadic diseases. It also contains an appended work concerning the anatomy of blood vessels, which is completely spurious. For this appended work is not consistent with actual observation, and is at odds with what is said in the second book of the *Epidemics*. Although after this it sets down those topics which were investigated in the book which I have already written about, still these things are noteworthy, well-expressed

---

53   Smith, 1979: 73–74.
54   *HNH*, Pref. CMG V 9,1, p. 7,19–21 Mewaldt (XV 9,15–16 K); Jouanna, 2012b: 320; Roselli, 2015: 534–535.

and concise, and adhere to the system of Hippocrates, as do also those things which are said concerning the healthy regimen.[55]

The context of this passage is the question of the authenticity of *On the Nature of Man* and *Regimen in Health*. Here we find some of Galen's criteria for authenticity, where he accepts or rejects parts of a treatise for different reasons. In the passage above, Galen talks about an appended work on blood vessels, which he rejects because it is not consistent with actual observation and it does not agree with a section in *Epidemics II*. Therefore, Galen is testing this passage on the basis of what he himself has seen from dissection, but also by comparison with another text from the Hippocratic writings. Galen trusts this particular section from *Epidemics II* as a standard that the passage from *On the Nature of Man* must be in agreement with to be authentic. Galen then tells us that his expectation is that the writing should be consistent with what he considers to be the style of writing of Hippocrates, using such terms as noteworthy (ἀξιόλογος) and concise (βραχύς). In addition, the content must also agree with what Galen calls the 'method' (τέχνη) of Hippocrates. This passage summarises Galen's criteria for the determination of the authenticity of Hippocratic works, which is based on two main factors; language (λέξις) and doctrine (διάνοια).

So in the passage above, we have Galen identifying the λέξις of part of this treatise as being consistent with what he expects of Hippocrates' writing style. Galen believed that in medical writing, language must be consistent and precise, utilising the best terminology. But, when the writing was aimed at a broad audience containing non-specialists, Galen was aware that some people may not be familiar with technical vocabulary of this kind. Therefore, there were some circumstances when Galen conceded that it might be necessary to distinguish between and explain the various terms more carefully for non-specialists.[56] But, correct usage of language is always paramount, as this provides secure understanding and avoids ambiguity.[57] In practice, Galen recommended that names be applied correctly according to the agreed conven-

---

55   ἔχει δὲ τὸν μὲν πρῶτον λόγον, ἔνθα περὶ τῶν στοιχείων καὶ τῶν χυμῶν διέρχεται, παντοίως ἐχόμε-
      νον τῆς Ἱπποκράτους τέχνης, ὥσπερ γε καὶ τὸν δεύτερον, ἔνθα καὶ τὰ διακριτικὰ τῶν ἐπιδημίων
      τε καὶ σποραδικῶν νοσημάτων. τὸν δὲ περὶ τῆς τῶν φλεβῶν ἀνατομῆς ἐναργῶς παρεγκείμενον
      ἔχει, μοχθηρὸν ὅλον· οὔτε γὰρ τοῖς φαινομένοις ὁμολογεῖ καὶ τοῖς ἐν τῷ δευτέρῳ τῶν Ἐπιδημιῶν
      εἰρημένοις μάχεται. τῶν δ' ἑξῆς τὰ μὲν παρέγκειται, περὶ ὧν ὅτ' ἐξηγούμεθά σοι τὸ βιβλίον ἀκρι-
      βωθήσεται, τὰ δέ ἐστιν ἀξιόλογα καὶ διὰ βραχέων καλῶς εἰρημένα καὶ τῆς Ἱπποκράτους ἐχόμενα
      τέχνης, ὥσπερ ὅσα περὶ τῆς ὑγιεινῆς διαίτης εἴρηται. *HNH*, Pref. CMG V 9,1, p. 8,9–18 Mewaldt
      (XV 10,18–11,11 K), translation by Lewis.
56   *Nat. Fac.* I (II 2,1–17 K).
57   See von Staden, 1995: 515.

tions in medical writing. Clarity was the key factor, as ordinary Greek language is permitted as long as the consistency is maintained.[58] However, we shall see that Galen is not always consistent in his own terminology when it comes to writing about black bile.[59] The other type of determination of authenticity based on διάνοια has two different aspects. The first is whether the treatise actually matches what Galen considers to be experiential evidence (e.g. from dissection) and this is what he believes Hippocrates would have concurred with. The other type of test for doctrine is when Galen compares the treatise in question with what he considers to be a model passage from another treatise (or a different part of the same treatise), which he has already identified as being authentic Hippocratic writing. We can see this in the above passage when Galen compares the description of the blood vessels with information from *Epidemics II*. This is also the case for content that refers to the humours; blood, phlegm, yellow bile and black bile, as Galen believed that Hippocrates had developed a four-humour system and so any authentic Hippocratic text must conform to this system.[60]

Galen considered Hippocrates to be not only an excellent physician, but also an accomplished writer. Therefore, Galen was looking out for any grammatical mistakes in the Hippocratic texts, as a way of determining authenticity. There were two main areas of grammar which Galen particularly focused on: barbarisms (βαρβαρισμός: sounding of words) and solecisms (σολοικισμός: meaning and construction of words).[61] When Galen analyses a text, he never reports what he considers as genuine writing by Hippocrates to contain such barbarisms. When it comes to solecisms, Galen is more relaxed, as he acknowledges that sometimes such mistakes do not distort the meaning to such an extent that understanding is lost. But this is only the case when there are not too many solecisms in a particular treatise that would then produce too much obscurity.[62] What we find is that the analysis of the construction of the language is used as an indication of authenticity by Galen. In the case of specific words used in the text, he is looking out for anachronisms that for him should not be present in Hippocrates' writing.[63] So we have Galen's criticism of

---

58   *MM* (X 43,3–44,8; 61,8–11; 62,4–6; 139,9–13 K); *Diff. Puls.* (VIII 493,3–497,12; 657,15–674,5 K). See Hankinson, 1994b: 170–175; Manetti, 2009: 159.

59   For example, see chapter 4, section 1 below.

60   See chapter 1, section 2 above.

61   *Hipp. Fract.* I.1 (XVIIIb 324,2–8 K); *Hipp. Aph.* v.62; VII.68 (XVIIb 865,14–18; XVIIIa 183,13–16 K); *Diff. Puls.* II.5 (VIII 587,8–11 K). See Sluiter, 1995: 522.

62   *Hipp. Aph.* VII.56; VII.58 (XVIIIa 167,4–9; 170,1–7 K). See Sluiter, 1995: 522–523 and 527–528.

63   A good example of Galen applying this type of analysis of authenticity to a specific text is in his *Commentary on Prorrhetic I*. This commentary is interesting, as it is a rare case

the style of language (λέξις), which might obscure the intended meaning. For Galen, this is not always accidental, as there are cases where he believes that the λέξις used by the author of *Prorrhetic I* is intentionally obscure: this is something that he believes Hippocrates would never do.[64] In parallel to this criticism of λέξις, Galen also analyses this treatise on the presentation of doctrine (διά-νοια). The main issue that Galen raises is that this author of *Prorrhetic I* has a tendency to refer to symptoms as if they occur all the time, when in fact they are infrequent. The opposite is also a problem, when there is a general case that is treated as something that is only applied to one condition. Galen explains that this type of mistake is due to this author not understanding the Hippocratic *Epidemics*, as this treatise tells us how to differentiate correctly between what is generally or particularly valid.[65] Here again, Galen is comparing one text (*Prorrhetic I*) with the content of other texts (for example, parts of the *Epidemics*), which he considers to be authentic. So, on the basis of λέξις and διάνοια, Galen is able to state what he considers to be authentic in the Hippocratic writings, thereby rejecting passages, or even whole books as inauthentic, which should be ignored when it comes to understanding Hippocrates' view of medicine.

---

of a line-by-line exegesis of a text that was not considered by Galen as worthy of being attributed to Hippocrates. Galen's commentaries were usually produced to provide interpretation and explanation of any uncertainty in the treatises that were considered to be genuine Hippocratic works, which were used to teach Hippocratic doctrine. The reason why Galen decided to write the *Commentary on Prorrhetic I*, after receiving requests for it, was due to his confidence that under his expert guidance he could explain and draw attention to the parts of this treatise that are useful. Galen is concerned about the lack of clarity in *Prorrhetic I*, in comparison to his expectation of Hippocrates' excellent writing style. For example, Galen emphasises the clarity of a genuine Hippocratic text such as *On Prognostic* in *Diff. Resp.* III.4 (VII 905,5–9 K) and *Hipp. Prorrh.* I.1, CMG V 9,2, p. 3,20–27 Diels (XVI 490,10–18 K). See Roselli, 2015: 538–540.

64 *Hipp. Prorrh.* III.16, CMG V 9,2, p. 128,1–5 Diels (XVI 749.16–750.5 K). In the case of this treatise, Galen is less relaxed about the presence of solecisms, as for him there are too many for the text to be considered worthy of Hippocrates, or a genuine work of the Hippocratic tradition. *Hipp. Prorrh.* I.4, CMG V 9,2, pp. 13,27–14,13 Diels (XVI 511,3–512,5 K). See Anastassiou and Irmer, 1997, volume II.1, p. 433; Roselli, 2015: 548 and Craik, 2015: 239.

65 For a general statement about the issues involving διάνοια, see *Hipp. Prorrh.* II.1, CMG V 9,2, p. 51,6–7 Diels (XVI 587,7–8 K). For an example of his criticism of a particular case being applied as a general rule, see *Hipp. Prorrh.* II.31; II.40, CMG V 9,2, pp. 79,14–15; 85,26 Diels (XVI 650,1–2; 663,6 K). For the opposite problem, where a general rule is only applied to a single case, see *Hipp. Prorrh.* II.38, CMG V 9,2, p. 83,9–19 Diels (XVI 658,3–15 K). Galen remarks on the correct way to determine general and particular cases in the *Epidemics* in *Hipp. Prorrh.* III.34; III.7, CMG V 9,2, pp. 147,22–27; 115,3–25 Diels (XVI 788,12–789,1; 723,10–725,3 K). See also Roselli, 2015: 554–556.

Therefore, we find that Galen was not only fully aware of the 'Hippocratic Question'; but that also he was engaged in his own answer to it. There are three categories of texts that Galen used to classify the authenticity of the various treatises in what we now consider to be the works of the Hippocratic Corpus. The first category contains those works that he believes can be attributed directly to Hippocrates. The second category contains the treatises that are in agreement with what Galen considers to be the views of Hippocrates, but that were written by his close followers such as Polybos. Lastly, there are those treatises that contain a large amount of material that is too far away from what he identifies as genuine Hippocratic writing. In general, Galen is not so concerned about the distinction between the first and second of these categories, as long as the text is consistent with what he considers as being the true διάνοια of Hippocrates, even if it is written by someone else.[66]

We have seen that Galen had referred to the list of Dioscurides' 'most genuine and most useful works': *Aphorisms,*[67] *Prognostic,*[68] *Epidemics I* and

---

66   Flemming, 2008: 342.

67   Galen attributes the majority of *Aphorisms* to Hippocrates, but denies authenticity to certain aphorisms throughout all the sections and in particular the ones at the very end of section seven. *Hipp. Aph.* VII Pref. (XVIIIa 101,1–10 K). See Manetti and Roselli, 1994: 1536–1538. Galen raises the problems associated with the final aphorisms at the end of section seven. He ends his commentary when he reaches the eighty-first aphorism of section seven, even though there are still another six after this one. This is because Galen believes that the *Aphorisms* has undergone an editing process by different commentators over time. *Hipp. Aph.* VII.81 (XVIIIa 194,7–12 K). See Smith, 1979: 129–130; Anastassiou and Irmer, 1997, volume II.1, pp. 58–59. This is an example of Galen analysing a treatise with comparison to what he considers to be genuine Hippocratic texts.

68   Galen considered *Prognostic* to be an excellent example of Hippocrates' use of brevity in language to convey complex medical information, which would normally require much more detailed explanation. Galen makes frequent remarks in this commentary to emphasise that this treatise is genuinely by Hippocrates. We find that he praises this work highly because he regards it as being the best form of Hippocratic λέξις. *Hipp. Prog.* I.1; I.4; III.6, CMG V 9,2 pp. 197,12–14; 205,5–8; 328,11–22 Heeg (XVIIIb 2,6–8; 15,16–16,4; 230,6–231,1 K). See Manetti and Roselli, 1994: 1538; Anastassiou and Irmer, 1997, volume II.1, p. 395; Craik, 2015: 235. However, despite this high praise for *Prognostic*, Galen still singles out a passage where he believes that there is room for doubt about the authenticity of a small part of the text. In the sixth section of *Prognostic* there is a passage concerning the different types of sweating that may benefit or harm a patient during acute cases of fever. Galen discusses this passage in his *Commentary on Prognostic* and is concerned that Hippocrates does not refer to critical days when discussing sweat anywhere else. Galen suggests that this error might be explained by an addition from the Hippocratic editors Artemidorus and Dioscurides. Hippocratic Corpus, *Prog.* VI (II 122,18–124,12 L); Galen, *Hipp. Prog.* I.26, CMG V 9,2 pp. 241,10–243,16 Heeg (XVIIIb 81,4–85,6 K). See Roselli, 2015: 534–535. Here Galen identifies a potentially inauthentic passage based on issues concerning what he

III,[69] *On Regimen in Acute Diseases*[70] and *Airs, Waters and Places.*[71] It is the case that all of these treatises were considered by Galen to be authentic and they are used by him as Hippocratic evidence to support his presentation of the characterisation of black bile. However, even in these treatises, there are cases where Galen questions the authenticity of single passages, or whole sections, which he suspects have been amended or even added in by some of the

---

considers to be the true writing of Hippocrates. It also allows him to reject short sections and passages from a work that he mostly regards as by Hippocrates. This flexibility is useful for Galen, as sometimes there are parts of treatises that may not be compatible with his view of what is and is not Hippocratic. Therefore, this allows him to ignore anything that he does not agree with or that may contradict his argument.

69   We find that *Epidemics I* and *III* were considered by Galen to be the oldest and most authentic works of Hippocrates. See Anastassiou and Irmer, 1997, volume II.1, pp. 174; 229–230, see also Mattern, 2008: 29.

70   The treatise *On Regimen in Acute Diseases* is generally presented as being divided into two parts. The first part is thought to be consistent with accepted Hippocratic writing, but the second part is considered to be of dubious authenticity and so has been designated as 'spurious' (νόθος). Modern naming of these texts follows this separation, for example using the abbreviated name of the first part: *Acut.*, and the second part: *Acut.* [*Sp.*]. However, sometimes the second part is named: *Acut.* [*Appendix*]. See Craik, 2015: 1. Galen rejects the Hippocratic authenticity of the last part of *On Regimen in Acute Diseases* (*Acut.* [*Sp.*]) because it is not worthy of the λέξις and διάνοια of Hippocrates. *HVA*, IV Pref. CMG V 9,1, pp. 271,9–11; 271,22–272,3 Helmreich (XV 733,2–4; 733,17–734,4 K). See Smith, 1979: 136–137; Anastassiou and Irmer, 1997, volume II.1, pp. 20–21; Craik, 2015: 4 and Roselli, 2015: 536–537. We find that, according to Galen, the first part was not published during Hippocrates' lifetime. This is because, although the content is consistent with the style and content of Hippocrates' writing, Galen considered the ordering of some of the passages to be different from what is found in genuine Hippocratic works. For example: *HVA*, II.55, CMG V 9,1, pp. 216,24–217,2 Helmreich (XV 624,5–625,14 K). See Anastassiou and Irmer, 1997, volume II.1, p. 2. He emphasises the authenticity of this first part in his commentaries on other Hippocratic texts, as he lists *On Regimen in Acute Diseases* alongside the other treatises that he considers to be authentic, such as *Prognostic* and *Epidemics I* and *III*. For example: *Hipp. Epid.* II, CMG V 10,1, pp. 275,31 f.; 402,17 Pfaff; *Hipp. Epid.* III.I.2, CMG V 10,2,1, p. 3,16–19 Wenkebach (XVIIa 484,13–16 K); *Hipp. Prog.* CMG V 9,2 p. 206,13–15 Heeg (XVIIIb 18,7–9 K). See Anastassiou and Irmer, 1997, volume II.1, p. 2. Galen makes a comparison between his own *On the Therapeutic Method* and the Hippocratic *On Regimen in Acute Diseases*, stating that from an educational view his own work is more complete and ordered than this Hippocratic work. But this does not mean that it is not genuine, just that Hippocrates cannot be expected to have completely systemised such a vast subject in medicine. *HVA*, II.36, CMG V 9,1, p. 196,13–17 Helmreich (XV 583,10–16 K). See Manetti and Roselli, 1994: 1542.

71   Galen attributes *Airs, Waters and Places* to Hippocrates, as being of the same high standard as the best examples of authentic treatises such as *On Prognostic*, *Aphorisms* and *Epidemics I* and *III*. For example, *Hipp. Aph.* III.11 (XVIIb 578,4–579,9; 582,18–584,6 K); *Hipp. Aer.* fol. 63v14–21. See Anastassiou and Irmer, 1997, volume II.1, pp. 26–27 and 38–40.

editors of the transmitted texts. In addition to these treatises, Galen also identified *On Humours*,[72] *On Diseases of Women I, II and III*,[73] *Koan Prognoses*,[74]

---

72   It seems likely that Galen considered *On Humours* to be a genuine work by Hippocrates.
     However, the *Commentary on On Humours* that had originally been attributed to Galen is
     itself now considered to be inauthentic. The version contained in the sixteenth volume
     of the Kühn collection of Galenic works has been identified as inauthentic, and may have
     been produced in the Renaissance period. The commentary that Galen wrote on the Hip-
     pocratic *On Humours* was composed of three books. There are a few references to this
     commentary in Galen's commentary on *Epidemics*: *Hipp. Epid.* III.1 CMG V 10,1, pp. 102,23–
     25; 108,24–25 Wenkebach (XVIIa 204,12–15; 215,16–18 K); III.2 Pref. CMG V 10,2,1, p. 61,11–13
     Wenkebach (XVIIa 578,4–7 K); *Lib. Prop.* 9 (XIX 35–36 K). See von Staden, 2006b: 138. How-
     ever, Galen's actual commentary is lost and only now survives in fragments. For more
     information on the commentary on *On Humours* in the Kühn Galenic collection that is
     considered to be a Renaissance forgery, see Deichgräber, 1972. More generally, see Manetti
     and Roselli, 1994: 1540; Anastassiou and Irmer, 1997, volume II.2, pp. xi–xii; Craik, 2015: 130.
     This commentary follows the same structure of the genuine commentaries by Galen, such
     as *Aphorisms*, as it contains a short preface and then a line-by-line exegesis of short sec-
     tions of the Hippocratic text in sequence from the very first sentence to the very last one in
     this treatise. There are sections of this commentary that contain information on material
     that represents Galen's elemental theory of health and disease. For example, near to the
     start there are references to the four-humour system of the Hippocratic *On the Nature of
     Man* in relation to the elements, qualities and humours, which is similar to Galen's *On the
     Elements According to Hippocrates*. In fact, this Galenic treatise is named as a source for
     further reading. See Pseudo-Galen, *Hipp. Hum.*, 1 XVI 4,11–61,10 K. Therefore, information
     on Galen's view of *On Humours* must be taken from what he says about this treatise in
     other works. The fact that Galen tells us that he had written a commentary on this trea-
     tise, and his frequent references to its passages, suggests that *On Humours* was part of the
     works that Galen identified as authentic Hippocratic treatises. The large amount of mate-
     rial that Galen references and quotes from this work, along with attribution of the content
     to Hippocrates, indicates that the style and content of the writing were of a standard com-
     parable to the other works that he considered as authentic. For example, see *HVA*, II.45,
     CMG V 9.1 p. 207,6–11 Helmreich (XV 604,13–16 K); *Hipp. Aph.* I.20; I.22; IV.4 (XVIIb 437,5;
     443,4; 663,9 K). For more examples see Anastassiou and Irmer, 1997, volume II.1, pp. 306–
     307 and II.2, p. 243; Garofalo, 2005: 445.
73   The three books under the title *On Diseases of Women* are a loosely connected collection of
     works. Galen refers to the third book of this series as *On Infertile Women* and we find that he
     draws frequently from the whole collection. Galen glosses a large amount of material from
     all three books and references passages from *On Diseases of Women I* in some of his trea-
     tises. See Anastassiou and Irmer, 1997, volume II.1, pp. 342–357 and 448–449; II.2 pp. 257;
     Craik, 2015: 204. Galen attributes all three books to Hippocrates, but it seems that they do
     not have the same status, when it comes to λέξις and διάνοια, as the best of Hippocrates'
     works such as *Prognostic, Aphorisms* and *Epidemics I* and *III*. *Hipp. Epid.* II, CMG V 10.1
     pp. 297,16–22 and 344,16–18 Pfaff; *Hipp. Aph.* IV.2; V.36; V.45 (XVIIb 660,3; 827,2; 838,12 K);
     Gloss. XIX 88,16; 105,8; 145,15 K. See Anastassiou and Irmer, 1997, volume II.1, pp. 341–342
     and 350.
74   We find that there are situations where Galen draws upon *Koan Prognoses*. For example,

On Breaths[75] and *On the Nature of Bones*[76] as authentic works by Hippocrates. Again, we find that Galen also points out the parts of these texts that he believes are not authentic. These treatises, although not part of Dioscurides' 'most gen-

---

there are some words and phrases from this treatise that are listed in Galen's *Glossary of Hippocratic Terms. Gloss.* XIX 69; 81 K. See Smith, 1979: 156–157 and Craik, 2015: 50. It seems that Galen regarded some parts of this treatise as being higher in quality, on the basis of λέξις and διάνοια, than other parts, as he lists the superior passages alongside what he considers to be the most genuine Hippocratic texts such as *On Prognostic, Aphorisms* and *Epidemics. Hipp. Epid.* (III.II) Pref. CMG V 10,2,1 p. 62,6–12 Wenkebach (XVIIa 578,18–579,8 K). See Anastassiou and Irmer, 1997, volume II.1, p. 167.

75 The question about the authorship of *On Breaths* is still open for debate, but there are some parallels between this treatise and other texts in the Hippocratic Corpus. For example, Craik refers to similarity with parts of *On the Nature of Man*, such as the removal or addition of key substances in the body and a distinction between two types of disease. See *Flat.* I and VI (90,2–92,15 and 96,20–98,13 L); *Nat. Hom.* 9, CMG I Jouanna (VI 52,4–56,12 K). Craik also discusses other examples, such as *On the Sacred Disease, On Fractures* and *On Diseases I.* See Craik, 2015: 100–101. From Galen's point of view, although he does not refer to this treatise by name in any of his extant writing, he does in fact refer to Hippocrates as the source of passages that he quotes from *On Breaths.* This indicates that at least some of this work was of a sufficiently high standard for Galen to attribute it directly to Hippocrates. For example, Galen names Hippocrates in quoted sections of *On Breaths* in *AA,* VIII.4 (II 674,9–15 K); *CAM,* II.2–3, CMG V 1,3, pp. 86,27–88,1 Fortuna (I 260,16–261,6 K) and *MM,* XI.9 (X 761,8–10 K). See Anastassiou and Irmer, 1997, volume II.2, pp. 224–225. One particular example is Galen's frequent use of 'opposites are the cure of opposites' (τὰ ἐναντία τῶν ἐναντίων ἐστὶν ἰήματα), which is found in *On Breaths. Flat.* I (VI 92,10–11 L). For Galen's many references to this passage see Anastassiou and Irmer, 1997, volume II.1, pp. 281–287 and volume II.2, pp. 225–227 and Lloyd, 1996: 268–269. Further to this, there is some similarity between the opening section of *On Breaths* and the beginning of Galen's *Commentary on Aphorisms* that might indicate that he has been influenced in his writing by the ideas contained in this treatise. Compare Hippocratic Corpus, *Flat.* I (VI 90,1–92,15 L) with Galen, *Hipp. Aph.* I.1 (XVIIb 354,2–355,3 K). See Craik: 2015: 102. There are also many other references by Galen that could be linked to parts of *On Breaths. HVA,* I.43, CMG V 9,1 p. 157,13–15 Helmreich (XV 502,1–4 K); *Hipp. Aph.* II.34 (XVIIb 530,14 K); *Hipp. Epid.* VI.II.9, CMG V 10,2,2 p. 69,13–15 Wenkebach (XVIIa 914,6–8 K); IV.27 p. 245,7 Pfaff; *Hipp. Off. Med.* III.33 (XVIIIb 906,12 K). See Anastassiou and Irmer, 1997, volume II.1, p. 281.

76 It is the case that Galen refers to some terms and passages from *On the Nature of Bones*, which indicates that he engaged with this treatise. For example, *Gloss.* XIX 114,2–3; 128,1–2 K. See Craik, 2015: 225. Sometimes Galen chooses to refer to this treatise under the title of *Leverage*, instead of *On the Nature of Bones. Hipp. Aer.* 93r14–94v4: "Hippocrates has mentioned these veins in his book, which is called *Leverage*, where he says:" (*Hippokrates hat diese Venen auch in seinem Buch erwähnt, das Mochlikon heisst, wo er sagt:*). See Anastassiou and Irmer, 1997, volume II.1, p. 45 and 391–392. However, it is difficult to tell exactly what Galen thinks about the standard of λέξις and διάνοια in this treatise. There are occasions when he clearly identifies Hippocrates as the source of some of the

uine and most useful works', are important for the understanding of the way that Galen characterises black bile and its role in producing disease in the body. Further to this, there are other important Hippocratic treatises that are missing from Dioscurides' list. For example, although *Airs, Waters and Places* is considered to be a very important genuine Hippocratic text, *On the Sacred Disease*, which contains similar material, is not listed and in general Galen seems to have ignored this treatise.[77] But, there is some very important material in *On the Sacred Disease*, which would be useful to support some of Galen's arguments involving the role of humours in the production of different types of disease. In addition to these 'most authentic' Hippocratic texts, there are also the treatises that Galen believes were not written by Hippocrates himself. However, they do contain material that is close enough to what he regards as the genuine works of Hippocrates. These are *Epidemics II, IV and VI*,[78] and *On Internal Affections*.[79] Therefore, in Galen's opinion, these treatises would be produced by

---

material from this treatise. However, in one particular case the content on anatomy in this treatise is close to the anatomy described in a section from *On the Nature of Man*, which Galen had identified as being inauthentic. Compare chapter nine of the Hippocratic *Oss.* (IX (IX 174,13–178,2 L)) with chapter eleven of the Hippocratic *Nat. Hom.* (11, CMG I 1,3, pp. 192,15–196,15 Jouanna (VI 58,1–60,19 L)) and Galen's *PHP* (VI.3.29, CMG V 4,1,2 p. 380,8–9 (V 528,12–14 K)). See Anastassiou and Irmer, 1997, volume II.2, p. 299.

77   Galen does refer to the title of *On the Sacred Disease* in his *Commentary on Joints*, and we find that he glosses a few of the terms present in this text. *Hipp. Artic.* 26 (XVIIIa 356,6–8 K); *Gloss.* XIX 74,6–8; 77,10; 127,8–10 and 152,11 K. See Anastassiou and Irmer, 1997, volume II.1, pp. 340–341. But, it is not clear exactly what Galen thought about the style and content of the writing in *On the Sacred Disease*, as he does not quote or reference material from this treatise in comparison to his many references to *Airs, Waters and Places*. There has been some discussion of the possibility that Galen rejected the authenticity of *On the Sacred Disease*. But, the evidence for this comes from a comment in a tenth century CE manuscript: Marcianus ven. gr. 269,84v. However, as Littré points out, we do not find this denial of authenticity in any of the extant writing by Galen. See Littré, 1961 (I): 353–354; Anastassiou and Irmer, 1997, volume II.2, p. 256.

78   The three books, *Epidemics II, IV* and *VI*, can be considered to be in the second category of authenticity, as Galen approves of their general content, but does not consider that they have the same level of λέξις that he expects from Hippocrates in *Epidemics I* and *III. Hipp. Epid.* II, CMG V 10,1, p. 302,38–43 Pfaff. See Anastassiou and Irmer, 1997, volume II.1, pp. 199–200; 241–242 and 248; Hanson, 1998: 33–34. For example, Galen tells us in his *Commentary on Epidemics VI* that there are variations in language, but not in the overall διάνοια that can be considered as being true to Hippocrates. *Hipp. Epid.* VI.1.2; VI.11.37; VI.11.47; VI.11.48; VI.IV.5; VI.V.36, CMG V 10,2,2, pp. 7,12–13; 104,16–20; 121,28–29; 123,11–14; 195,12–14; 320,13 Wenkebach (XVIIa 800,12–13; 975,17–976,4; 1006,2–3; 1008,11–15; XVIIb 131,7–9; 310,5–6 K). See Roselli, 2015: 537.

79   It seems that Galen knew about *On Internal Affections*, as part of a larger work with the

Hippocrates' closest associates. This allows Galen to draw upon these works as being Hippocratic, but he has even more flexibility to reject parts of them, if he feels that they are not in agreement with a particular argument or a point that he is making. Finally, there are the treatises that Galen either explicitly rejected as being by Hippocrates or Hippocratic, or ones about which he is completely silent. These are *Epidemics V and VII*,[80] *On Diseases I–III*,[81] *On Diseases IV*,[82]

more general title *On Affections. Hipp. Aph.* VI.27 (XVIIIa 39,1–4 K); *Hipp. Artic.* 18 (XVIIIa 512,15–16 K). See Anastassiou and Irmer, 1997, volume II.1, pp. 313–314. Galen, in agreement with the general opinion of this treatise at the time, considered *On Internal Affections* to be part of a set of what were known as Hippocratic works on the study of diseases. However, these texts were later than the ones that he considered to be written by Hippocrates himself. Therefore, this text comes under the category of being close enough in style and content for Galen to consider it to be a Hippocratic work. Craik, 2015: 136.

80 Galen rejected *Epidemics V* and *VII* as inauthentic on the basis of what he considered to be proper Hippocratic λέξις and διάνοια. For *Epidemics V*, see *Hipp. Epid.* II, CMG V 10,1, pp. 310,41–311,2; 350,13 Pfaff; *Hipp. Epid.* (VI) Pref. CMG V 10,2,2, p. 5,8 Wenkebach (XVIIa 796,8 K). See also Anastassiou and Irmer, 1997, volume II.1, pp. 244–245. For *Epidemics VII*, see *Hipp. Epid.* (VI) Pref.; VI.III.14; VI.III.15 CMG V 10,2,2 pp. 5,8; 144,15–16; 146,7–8 Wenkebach (XVIIa 796,8; XVIIb 39,5–6; 42,6–8 K). See also Anastassiou and Irmer, 1997, volume II.1, p. 277; Hanson, 1998: 33–34.

81 The first three books of *On Diseases* do not follow a sequential pattern and so are not considered to be linked in the way that their naming suggests. Craik, 2015: 169. The same is true for *On Diseases IV*. However, Galen did know about the existence of these books and refers to what we now call *Diseases I* as *On the Cases of Purulence. Hipp. Artic.* 18 (XVIIIa 512,15–513,5 K); *HVA*, II.38; III.15, CMG V 9.1 pp. 198,3–6; 237,4–7 Helmreich (XV 587,5–8; 663,17–664,2 K). See Smith, 1979: 127; Anastassiou and Irmer, 1997, volume II.1, p. 328 and Craik, 2015: 170. He has a negative attitude to material from these three books of *On Diseases* and he does not consider them to be genuine Hippocratic works. Anastassiou and Irmer, 1997, volume II.1, pp. 328–329. We have already seen that Galen reports that there were some ancient writers who attributed *On Diseases II* to Hippocrates (the son of Thessalos), who was a grandson of the great Hippocrates, although Galen does not support this theory himself (see page 37 above). Therefore, from the lack of any positive statement by Galen on the Hippocratic authenticity of *On Diseases I, II* and *III*, alongside the absence of these books in his listing of the best examples of genuine Hippocratic texts (for example see *Prognostic*, see page 44 above) and no commentary by him, I will regard all three books from *On Diseases* as being considered inauthentic by Galen.

82 The traditional view of *On Diseases IV* was that it should be considered as part of a set of three integrated treatises with *On Generation* and *On the Nature of the Child*. However, Craik has argued against this grouping, and offers an alternative view of *On Diseases IV*. She suggests that, although *On Diseases IV* may be by the same author as *On Generation* and *On the Nature of the Child*, it should not be regarded as part of a close sequential set with these two treatises. Craik, 2015: 117 and 187. There is no explicit statement by Galen regarding this treatise, but it is likely that he would not have considered this text to be a genuine Hippocratic work.

On Places in Man[83] and *Ancient Medicine*.[84] I have included these treatises for two reasons. Firstly, there are the texts that contain material on black bile that is comparable to Galen's characterisation of this humour. Secondly, there are other texts, which do not contain any material on black bile, but offer alternative theories that are useful for comparison with Galen's biological system. This is important as it helps us to understand more about how and why Galen wrote about black bile. However, the most significant omission in Galen's writing on black bile from Dioscurides' list is *On the Nature of Man*. We have seen that this treatise was essential for Galen's presentation of Hippocrates' four-humour system and to some of his arguments relating to Hippocrates' status as a physician-philosopher. Therefore, it is important for Galen to include *On the Nature of Man* as one of the genuine Hippocratic works, so what does he say about the authenticity of this treatise?

When it comes to black bile, *On the Nature of Man* is the main treatise in the Hippocratic Corpus that presents this substance as part of a set of four fundamental fluids, which have become known as the four humours. In addition to the text of *On the Nature of Man* itself, there is an associated treatise called *On Regimen in Health*. However, there is a question over whether *On Regimen*

---

83   Galen does not attribute *On Places in Man* to Hippocrates or the related Hippocratic tradition that followed his doctrine. However, he does acknowledge that this work is one of the older books from the development of scientific writing in the fifth century BCE. *Hipp. Epid.* VI.II.9, CMG V 10,2,2 p. 67,1–12 Wenkebach (XVIIa 909,12–910,9 K). In Galen's *Commentary on Airs, Waters and Places* (91v7–92r6), he says: "Although this book does not belong to the authentic and unadulterated writings of Hippocrates, so we have no doubt but that it comes from one of the old scientists." (*Denn obwohl dieses Buch nicht zu den authentischen und unverfälschten Schriften des Hippokrates gehört, so zweifeln wir doch nicht, dass es von einem der alten Wissenschaftler stammt.*) See Anastassiou and Irmer, 1997, volume II.1, pp. 322–333. Galen's general view of the inauthenticity of *On Places in Man* is not always applied throughout his writing. For example, he makes frequent citations to passages and terms from this work and sometimes attributes them to Hippocrates, but he does not actually name this text. See Anastassiou and Irmer, 1997, volume II.2, pp. 249–250. See also Craik, 2015: 161.

84   In ancient times, there were some commentators who considered this treatise to be written by Hippocrates. For example, Erotian, *vocum Hippocraticum collectio*, 38,6–9; 40,4–6; 130,11–13. See Anastassiou and Irmer, 1997, volume I, pp. 458–459. Littré has attempted to support the authenticity of *Ancient Medicine* by suggesting that the twentieth chapter of this work is the source for Plato's writing on Hippocrates' methodology in the *Phaedrus* (270c–e). See Jones, 1923a: 3–9; Littré, 1961 (I): 294–296; Craik, 2015: 284. In contrast, Galen was not impressed with *Ancient Medicine* and did not consider it an authentic Hippocratic work. He did not think that the material presented in this work was consistent with what he believes was developed by Hippocrates and those that followed true Hippocratic doctrine. Craik, 2015: 284–285.

in Health should be regarded as part of *On the Nature of Man*, or as a separate work in its own right.[85] Galen's view was that these two works should be considered as separate treatises, as he wrote a separate commentary on *On Regimen in Health*. But, I am going to discuss *On Regimen in Health* alongside *On the Nature of Man* in this section, as Galen engaged with the debate about the authorship of both these treatises, and argued for a solution that divides *On the Nature of Man* into two distinct parts, with *On Regimen in Health* regarded as a separate work. He names Hippocrates as the originator of the first eight chapters of *On the Nature of Man*, but concedes that *On Regimen in Health* may have been written by Polybos. However, he denies Hippocratic authenticity to chapters nine to fifteen of *On the Nature of Man*, suggesting instead that these were written by a forger who wanted to create a larger volume to impress the Attalid and Ptolemaic kings, who put a higher price on longer works.[86] In Galen's opinion, the first eight chapters of *On the Nature of Man* contain key Hippocratic διά-νοια, such as the proper mixture or separation of the four humours to explain the causes of health and disease.[87] We have seen already (see pages 40–41 above) that in his *Commentary on On the Nature of Man*, Galen quotes his (lost) work *The Authentic and Spurious Writings of Hippocrates* on this very issue concerning the authenticity of this treatise. A little later in this commentary, he attempts to strengthen his argument by connecting a passage in the *Phaedrus* with the first eight chapters of *On the Nature of Man*. This association provides an example of Plato's description of Hippocrates' methodology for medicine.[88] However, when it comes to *On Regimen in Health*, he judges this text to be close enough in writing style and content to be a Hippocratic treatise, but not necessarily written by Hippocrates himself.[89]

Galen concedes that it is possible that the author of *On Regimen in Health* might have been Polybos. But, he is adamant that chapters nine to fifteen of *On the Nature of Man* cannot possibly be attributed to Hippocrates, or even to

---

85   Craik points to the difference of opinion in modern scholarship, where we have both Littré and Jones regarding them as two separate works and Jouanna combining them in his 1975 translation and commentary. For more information on this debate, see Jones, 1931: xxvi–xxvii; Littré, 1962 (VI): 70; Jouanna, 2002a: 20–21; Craik, 2015:208–209.

86   *HNH*, II Pref. CMG V 9,1, p. 57,4–21 Mewaldt (XV 108,4–109,17 K); *Hipp. Vict.* Pref. CMG V 9,1, p. 89,3–14 Mewaldt (XV 174,5–175,9 K). See Smith, 1979: 166–172; 201–202 and 219–221; Hanson, 1998: 33; Jouanna, 2012b: 320–321 and Craik, 2015: 208–209.

87   *HNH*, Pref. CMG V 9,1, pp. 6,6–7,21 Mewaldt (XV 7,4–9,16 K). See Smith, 1979: 170; Jouanna, 2012b: 314 and 333.

88   Plato, *Phdr.* 270c–d; Galen, *HNH*, Pref. CMG V 9.1, pp. 8,19–9,11 Mewaldt (XV 11,11–13,4 K).

89   *Hipp. Vict.* Pref. CMG V 9,1, p. 89,3–14 Mewaldt (XV 174,5–175,9 K). See Flemming, 2008: 341; Jouanna, 2012b: 315 and 324.

one of his close associates, such as Polybos. At the end of his *Commentary on On the Nature of Man*, Galen accuses Sabinus and 'most of the exegetes' (τῶν πλείστων ἐξηγητῶν) of first praising these seven chapters and then claiming that the author was Polybos. Galen criticises them for believing that a Hippocratean, like Polybos, could have written the material in these chapters of *On the Nature of Man*, as, according to Galen, the information in this section does not correspond to Hippocratic writing.[90] For example, in chapter nine of *On the Nature of Man* there is a section on diseases that are caused by repletion (πλησμονή) in the body. Galen acknowledges that some diseases arise from this type of repletion, but says that this is not necessarily the underlying cause of the disease. Galen defines disease as a certain condition that harms the function of the body. Therefore, he does not believe that repletion alone is harmful, but instead it causes harm through some intermediary condition. Furthermore, repletion can be defined in two ways. The first is as a fundamental property and the second is as the capacity of a vessel. We are told that the former causes the humours to be corrupt and will tend to send a humour to the weakest part of the body. The latter causes the vessels in the body to rupture and can be fatal due to the blockage of the body's transpirations. But Galen says that the writer of this part of *On the Nature of Man* is incorrect in using repletion to counteract the draining of humours in the body. Galen's view is that all Greeks know that repletion is applied to excesses of a well-balanced quality. In this case the humours are emptying and so rebalance cannot be produced by repletion. In addition, there are some doctors who do not use the draining of humours as the cause of disease; instead they reserve this term to describe the weakening of the body. However, Galen counters this argument with the statement that diseases do arise from imbalanced draining, as this causes a cooling effect and can produce fever.[91] These are examples of Galen's argument that this part of *On the Nature of Man* cannot be by Hippocrates or someone following Hippocratic doctrine.

Another example that Galen provides to reject this section of *On the Nature of Man* is the content referring to blood vessels. The problem is that, in the eleventh chapter of *On the Nature of Man*, we are told that there are four pairs of the major blood vessels in the body. Galen says that this is a clear error that Hippocrates (or a close follower like Polybos) would not make. Furthermore, it is inconsistent with *Epidemics II*, which Galen acknowledges as containing

---

90   *HNH*, II.22, CMG V 9,1, pp. 87,15–88,13 Mewaldt (XV 171,9–172,14 K). See Smith, 1979: 171; Manetti and Roselli, 1994: 1555–1556.

91   Hippocratic Corpus, *Nat. Hom.* 9, CMG I 1,3, p. 188,3–6 Jouanna (VI 52,4–7 L); Galen, *HNH*, II.1, CMG V 9,1, pp. 58,15–59,12 Mewaldt (XV 111,3–114,10 K).

proper Hippocratic doctrine (see page 48 above). In this way, Galen is writing against the view of Aristotle, who quotes this passage on blood vessels in *On the History of Animals* and attributes it to Polybos. The issue here concerns correct knowledge about the inner structure of the body and Galen defends Hippocrates' general presentation of anatomy, saying that he did not need to provide a lot of detail at this time. However, the information he does present is correct and so this is why this section cannot be attributed to Hippocrates or one of his close followers.[92] This is another example where Galen makes a decision on authenticity based on διάνοια, which he analyses from both the point of view of general medical knowledge that he believes that Hippocrates would agree with, and from a passage in another text from the Hippocratic writings that he has identified as being genuine.

A further example comes from the fifteenth chapter of *On the Nature of Man*, where quotidian fevers are said to be of less duration than tertian. Galen points out that this is inconsistent with *Epidemics I* and *Aphorisms*, both of which he considers to be examples of genuine works by Hippocrates.[93] It is Galen's opinion that a physician who believes that the quotidian fever reaches a crisis in a shorter time than the tertian is not very skilled in medicine. But Galen does not say that this part of *On the Nature of Man* has been written intentionally as a lie. Instead, this has been constructed from a theory, which associates constant fevers with an excess of fire, quotidian to air, tertian to water and quartan to the earth. Galen cites a passage in Plato's *Timaeus* as representing this view.[94] Galen then puts forward what he believes to be the most plausible account. The origin of the different fevers is due to the hot element and the difference between the fevers is due to the amount of heat that they contain. So the most constant fever contains the most fire, and then as the gap between the bouts of fever increases, the temperature is reduced.[95] This issue of the inconsistency of the cause of the different fevers in *On the Nature of Man* has been blamed by commentators, such as Sabinus, on Polybos being mistaken when writing this text. Sabinus has assumed that Polybos did not have access to *Epidemics I* and

---

92   Aristotle, *HA*, III.3, 512b13–513a8. See Lloyd, 1993: 131; Nutton, 2004: 85; Jouanna, 2012b: 314–315. Jouanna argues that Galen's failure to acknowledge Aristotle's quotation of this passage in *On the History of Animals* and his attribution of it to Polybos threatens Galen's argument against the authenticity of this middle section of *On the Nature of Man*. See Jouanna, 2012b: 322–323.

93   Hippocratic Corpus, *Nat. Hom.* 15, CMG I 1,3, pp. 202,10–204,21 Jouanna (VI 66,10–68,16 L); cf. *Aph.* IV.59 (IV 522,15–16 L); Galen, *HNH*, II.22, CMG V 9,1, pp. 85,18–86,4 Mewaldt (XV 167,16–169,1 K). See Smith, 1979: 171.

94   Plato, *Ti.*, 86a; Galen, *HNH*, II.22, CMG V 9,1, p. 86,4–24 Mewaldt (XV 169,1–170,6 K).

95   *HNH*, II.22, CMG V 9,1, pp. 86,25–87,14 Mewaldt (XV 170,6–171,9 K).

Aphorisms. But Galen does not think that the writer of this part of *On the Nature of Man* was a close follower of Hippocrates, as the author calls the 'continuous (συνεχής) fever' the 'non-intermittent (σύνοχος) fever', which Galen believes Hippocrates would never have done. Galen explains this as a more recent term used by physicians, who do not know about the different terminology used by the ancient authors.[96] So again we find that Galen has questioned the authenticity of a part of a treatise based on διάνοια from what he considers as correct knowledge of medicine and by reference to other texts in the Hippocratic Corpus, which contradict this material, but are considered by him as authentic. This shows that Galen is willing to go against a traditional view of the authorship of *On the Nature of Man*, even if this contradicts the writing of Aristotle and Plato. This treatise is important to Galen, as the first eight chapters contain material on the four-humour system, but he is willing to reject some parts of this work as not being authentic, as they do not fit into his own view of what constitutes the correct διάνοια of Hippocrates on issues concerning aetiology of disease and information on anatomy.

The majority of the references to black bile are in the first eight chapters of *On the Nature of Man*, which, according to Galen, correspond to the section of this treatise that is genuinely by Hippocrates. The importance of this content for Galen is demonstrated by his use of this material to present what he believes is a theory created by Hippocrates and also to support his own biological theory of the body that draws upon the theory of the four humours.[97] We find that black bile is referred to in chapters nine to fifteen of *On the Nature of Man*,

---

96   Hippocratic Corpus, *Nat. Hom.* 15, CMG I 1,3, pp. 202,10–204,21 Jouanna (VI 66,10–68,16 L); Galen, *HNH*, II.22, CMG V 9,1, pp. 87,14–88,13 Mewaldt (XV 171,9–173,4 K). However, as Roselli has argued, this method is not robust enough to reject this type of language, as other Hippocratic writing suggests that this was an acceptable Ionic form for this time period. See Roselli, 2015: 537.

97   For example, *Nat. Hom.* 4–7, CMG I 1,3, pp. 172,13–15; 174,12–176,1; 176,13–178,1; 180,3–7; 182,8–9; 184,13–14 and 186,8–9 Jouanna (VI 38,19–40,2; 40,16–17; 42,12–14; 44,14–15; 44,17–18; 46,13–14; 48,16–17 and 50,7–9 L). Galen makes frequent reference to this material on the humours and black bile throughout his writing. For section IV: *Hipp. Elem.* 10.1–3, CMG V 1,2, pp. 138,15–140,1 De Lacy (I 492,1–10 K); *Prop. Plac.* 12.5, CMG V 3,2, p. 98,5–7 Nutton; *At. Bil.* 5; 6, CMG V 4,1,1, pp. 79,1–24; 83,20–24 De Boer (V 119,14–121,10; 128,6–10 K); *PHP*, VIII.4.13–17; 24; 6.1–14, CMG V 4,1,2, pp. 500,26–502,9; 504,3–15; 512,25–516,6 De Lacy (V 674,14–675,17; 677,6–678,4; 689,1–692,12 K). For section V: *HNH*, I.28, CMG V 9,1, p. 37,12–27 Mewaldt (XV 69,8–70,10 K); *Adv. Iul.* 8.9–10, CMG V 10,3, p. 65,14–21 Wenkebach (XVIIIa 292,8–293,1 K); *PHP*, VIII.5.26–39, CMG V 4,1,2, pp. 510,8–512,24 De Lacy (V 685,8–688,17 K). For section VI: *At. Bil.* 7, CMG V 4,1,1, p. 87,10–15 De Boer (V 135,13–136,1 K); *Hipp. Elem.* 13.12–16, CMG V 1,2, p. 152,4–15 De Lacy (I 503,17–504,14 K); *SMT*, III.27 (XI 616,11–14 K); *Purg. Med. Fac.* II (XI 330,7–14 K). For section VII: *Hipp. Epid.* III.I.6, CMG V 10,2,1, pp. 32,25–33,3 Wenkebach (XVIIa 534,14–17 K); *Hipp. Epid.* II, CMG V 10,1, pp. 4,13–5,25 Pfaff; *HNH*, I.37;

which Galen rejects as being Hippocratic. In the fifteenth chapter, the types of fever are discussed in relation to yellow bile and black bile. The cause of the quartan fever is related to the properties and nature of the black bile humour. Galen's rejection of this material is shown by the absence of any direct reference to this material in the presentation of his biological theory of the body, which is in contrast to his frequent use of the first eight chapters of this treatise.[98] When it comes to *On Regimen in Health*, there are no references to black bile at all.[99] This might be one of the reasons for Galen's lack of interest in *On Regimen in Health*, as it does not contain any important information on the humours, compared with the first eight chapters of *On the Nature of Man*. But, it is not sufficiently different in λέξις and διάνοια for Galen to reject it completely, as he does with chapters nine to fifteen of *On the Nature of Man*. Whatever his reasons, the way that Galen engages and makes decisions on the ideas contained in *On the Nature of Man* and *On Regimen in Health*, shows how he is selective in the material that he considers as either Hippocratic or inauthentic in relation to his own judgement on what constitutes the proper style and content of Hippocrates' writing.

4   Galen's Polemic against Those He Considers to be Opposed to Humoral Theory

The last major influence I want to discuss in this chapter is Galen's engagement in rhetoric and polemic against rival physicians and philosophers. In contrast to those that Galen considered to be Hippocratic humoral theorists, we also find that he was very critical of anyone who denied the importance or existence of the humours in relation to health and disease in the body. For example, in *On the Doctrines of Hippocrates and Plato*, Galen claims that Erasistratus rejected the idea of an association between the four humours and the four elemental qualities.[100] Further to this, in *On the Natural Faculties*, Galen complains that Erasistratus is ignorant of the 'genesis of the humours' (περὶ τῆς γενέσεως τῶν χυμῶν), as he does not say anything plausible about this subject.[101] For example,

---

CMG V 9,1, p. 46,5–11; 24–31 Mewaldt (XV 87,1–9; 88,5–13 K); *Temp.* II.3; III.4 (I 603,7–14; 673,11–674,1 K). See Anastassiou and Irmer, 1997, volume II.1, pp. 362–365 and volume II.2, pp. 269–279.

98   *Nat. Hom.* 15, CMG I 1,3, p. 204,12–19 Jouanna (VI 68,6–14 L).

99   There is a passage that refers to the purging of phlegm in winter and bile when the body is hot, see *Salubr.* V (VI 78,3–11 L).

100 *PHP*, VIII.5.25, CMG V 4,1,2, p. 510,5–8 De Lacy (V 685,4–8 K).

101 *Nat. Fac.* II.8; II.9 (II 107,4–10; 113,14–116,8; 141,16–142,3 K). See Vegetti, 1999b: 390–394.

in *On Black Bile* Galen admits that Erasistratus correctly connects the presence
of too much bile in the body as a cause of a type of jaundice, but points out
that it is also important to know whether this bile has come from food that contains a large amount of bile or that this bile has been generated in the body by
some process.[102] Galen also accuses Erasistratus of a neglect of the humours
in *On Affected Parts* and *On Black Bile*.[103] More generally, in texts such as *On
the Therapeutic Method*, Galen interprets Erasistratus' aetiology as being based
on 'proximate elements', which are the uniform parts of the body. This includes
substances such as blood, phlegm and yellow bile. It is not clear, as Leith points
out, exactly what Erasistratus postulated as the primary elements of the cosmos. But, it is likely that it may be similar to Aristotle's view of the qualities
and elements.[104] We find that Erasistratus acknowledged some aspects of the
importance of the humours in medicine, considering them to be pathogenic
substances that cause disease either by inhibiting the flow of other fluids in
certain places in the body, or by being in excess.[105] However, Galen reports
that Erasistratus did not write anything about black bile, and denies that black
bile is the cause of the melancholy illness or other diseases, such as cancer
and elephantiasis.[106] It is within this polemical context that Galen defends the
existence, status and function of black bile to explain health and disease in his
treatise *On Black Bile*.

Galen makes a similar criticism of the second century BCE physician, Asclepiades of Bithynia, in relation to his rejection of the four-humour system of *On
the Nature of Man*. For example, in *On the Elements According to Hippocrates*
and *On the Natural Faculties*, Galen attacks the corpuscular theory of Asclepiades, claiming that it is inferior to Hippocrates' theory because it cannot
account for the purgation of the four humours.[107] Asclepiades developed a
physiological theory, which proposed that certain fundamental particles, called
corpuscles (ἄναρμοι ὄγκοι), travel through the body. The proper balance of these
particles in the body promoted good health, but anything that might inhibit

---

102   *At. Bil.* 5, CMG V 4,1,1, pp. 80,26–81,9 De Boer (V 123,8–124,4 K).
103   *Loc. Aff.* III.10 (VIII 191,12–14 K). In *At. Bil.* (5; 7; 8, CMG V 4,1,1, pp. 82,3–5; 85,19–20; 88,6–
      7; 91,24–25 De Boer (V 125,13–15; 132,5–6; 137,7–8; 144,2–3 K)), Galen says that Erasistratus
      believed that speculation on the humours was useless and wrote nothing about the origins
      of the humours. See Jouanna, 2006: 119.
104   *MM*, II.5 (X 107,3–14 K). See Leith, 2015a: 464–470.
105   Nutton, 2004: 135–137; 2005: 118. Jouanna, 2006: 119.
106   *At. Bil.* 5; 7, CMG V 4,1,1, pp. 80,26–82,7; 85,19–86,10 De Boer (V 123,8–125,17; 132,5–133,13 K).
107   *Hipp. Elem.* 12.9–13.23, CMG V 1,2, pp. 148,5–154,10 De Lacy (I 500,16–506,7 K); *Nat. Fac.* I.13
      (II 43,15–44,12 K).

their movement could cause disease.[108] In this theory, the invisible corpuscles can, at certain times, clump together and block the invisible pores throughout the body, which normally allow the passage of the corpuscles. Alternatively, if the corpuscles become abnormally separated, then the body experiences relaxation. There has been some suggestion that in Galen's writing about Asclepiades' theory of matter, he associates Asclepiades with the Methodist school of medicine. However, Leith argues that there is no evidence that the Methodists postulated a doctrine relating to the 'void', which we find in Asclepiades' theory.[109] What we find is that Galen opposes Asclepiades' theory of matter because he believes that it cannot explain how pain can be felt in the body.[110] He also challenges Asclepiades concerning his views on the humours. For example, in *On the Natural Faculties*, Galen's view is that Asclepiades has disregarded what should be acknowledged as the true faculties in the body, and has developed an atomist theory, which fails to explain the most basic biological principles such as how blood is produced. There is further criticism of Asclepiades' ideas about the production of the humours. According to Galen, Asclepiades postulated that yellow bile is produced in the bile-ducts. In the case of drugs that purge humours, he also claims that Asclepiades believed that the humours are actually produced by the purgative drugs themselves. The outcome of this is that it does not matter which purgative drug is used for a treatment of any specific disease. This is because Asclepiades claimed that all purgative drugs will cleanse the body equally. One example given by Galen is the use of scammony to evacuate bile in the case of jaundice. We find that Asclepiades' theory would predict that this drug will actually turn blood into bile, harming the body. But Galen says that many people have been treated successfully with this drug. He warns that those who follow Asclepiades' theory

---

108　Leith provides a summary of the debate in modern scholarship on the question of Epicurean influence on Asclepiades' theory. Vallance has argued for Asclepiades' theory being closer to that of Erasistratus than the Epicureans. In opposition to this, Pigeaud and Casadei assert the Epicurean influence on Asclepiades' theory. Leith observes that the situation concerning Asclepiades' work cannot be explained by this polarised view. However, as Leith points out, the work of Polito shows that Asclepiades should be considered 'as an independent and innovative thinker'. This means that it is important to view Asclepiades' theory in relation to Epicurean atomism. Therefore, his association with this particular philosophical theory is more complex than it at first may seem. See Pigeaud, 1980: 176–200; 1981: 141; Furley and Wilkie (1984): 38–39; Vallance, 1990: 1, 10 and 123–130; Polito, 2006: 285–335; Leith, 2009: 284; 2012: 164–165.

109　*Caus. Morb.* 1; 7 (VII 1,1–2,14; 32,17–33,4 K); *SMT*, XI 783,7–12 K; *MM*, IV (X 267,14–268,6 K). See Frede, 1987: 272; Vallance, 1990: 57–58; Pellegrin, 2009: 676; Leith, 2012: 168–170.

110　*CAM*, VII.13, CMG V 1,3, p. 76,19–23 Fortuna (I 249,13–250,2 K). See Leith, 2009: 292.

will eventually start distrusting their own senses, when they make observations in these types of cases.[111] In addition to this, in *On the Elements According to Hippocrates*, Galen attacks Asclepiades on the inadequacy of his corpuscular theory to explain the purgation of the humours, as opposed to what he considers to be the best explanation in the Hippocratic *On the Nature of Man*.[112] Again, as in the case of Erasistratus, Galen believes that it is necessary to defend the status of black bile against rival theories in which this humour is either not considered to be a fundamental 'element' of the body, or does not exist at all.

5   Summary

Here we have seen that there are three important factors that have influenced the way that Galen writes about black bile. Firstly, Galen has emphasised the importance of philosophy in the development of a logically constructed theory in medicine. In this way, Galen attempts to connect the writing of Hippocrates on material relating to fundamental substances in the body with the work of philosophers, such as Plato and Aristotle. Galen also includes the type of teleology that we find in the writing of Plato and Aristotle, as being consistent with his interpretation of parts of the Hippocratic writings that he presents as having a teleological basis. We will see later in this book that Galen uses this type of doxographical argument to connect certain parts of the Hippocratic treatises with the work of philosophers, such as Plato and Aristotle in the development of his ideas concerning black bile. Galen goes further to suggest that Hippocrates was the originator of these ideas and that later physicians and philosophers followed on from Hippocrates' work. Secondly, we can see

---

111   *Nat. Fac.* I.13 (II 39,4–43,15 K). I will be going into more detail about Galen's criticism of Asclepiades' views on black bile and the spleen in chapter 6, section 3 below.

112   Galen tells us that Asclepiades' concept of nature, which is based on particles and pores, is contrary to all that is excellent in the art of medicine. Galen says that Hippocrates and all subsequent physicians have learned about the nature of purgative drugs by experience and testing. Galen asks the question, if purging is only beneficial because it empties the body, then why not open a vein and bleed a person, whatever the ailment? So, Asclepiades is forced into to his conclusion concerning purging because of the way that his particles and pores must operate in practice. There is the observation that when each drug draws out a specific humour, we find that further purgation is possible. According to Asclepiades' theory, during any purgation of the four humours, one of two things should have occurred; either the purging of a humour should cease, or only the first humour that is purged should be extracted. But neither of these is in agreement with observation. See *Hipp. Elem.* 12.1–2; 12.7–8; 13.16–19, CMG V 1,2, pp. 146,8–14; 146,23–148,4; 152,13–23 De Lacy (I 499,1–9; 500,5–16; 504,14–8 K). See also Pendrick, 1994: 227.

that Galen was influenced by some of his teachers, particularly in the case of
those whose own work focused on the Hippocratic treatises. We have seen evidence that Galen was in agreement with Dioscurides' list of the most genuine
Hippocratic treatises, which he used as the basis for his work on black bile as
a humour of the body. However, the treatise *On the Nature of Man* is not contained in this list and this text seems at best to be attributed to a Hippocratic
writer, such as Polybos, rather than by the Hippocrates himself. This has conse-
quences for Galen, as by selecting the humoral theory of *On the Nature of Man*
as the best explanation of health and disease in the body, along with identifying other texts in the Hippocratic writings as being genuine, he is implying
that there is agreement on the four-humour system on the basis of common
authorship of these treatises. This is particularly problematic in the treatises
that do not contain any material on black bile at all. The third major influence
on Galen's writing identified in this chapter is the way that Galen constructs his
rhetorical and polemical arguments against the views of his rivals, most importantly, the Erasistrateans and the followers of Asclepiades. We can see that the
existence and importance of the humours for the understanding of health and
disease was a particular point of disagreement between Galen and the views
of these two specific groups. Galen seems to feel that the case for black bile
needs to be defended against alternative theories of health and disease. It is
within these arguments that we need to understand what Galen has written
about black bile and how this affects the way he writes about this substance
in different contexts both within and between the Galenic treatises that have
survived.

CHAPTER 3

Galen's Qualitative and Structural Characterisation of Black Bile

In this chapter I will analyse Galen's characterisation of the physical and qualitative properties of black bile. This is important for our understanding about how and why Galen writes about black bile, as when it comes to the actual practice of medicine, we shall see that Galen stresses the need for a physician to be able to identify substances correctly in order to properly diagnose an illness.

1   The Essential Properties of Black Bile

There are a number of characteristics that can be used to identify different substances based on their appearance and how they feel when touched. I am going to start with the way that black bile is characterised on the basis of the four qualities, hot, cold, dry and wet, as they represent the most basic properties that affect the body.[1] For example, in *On Mixtures*, they are presented as being the most fundamental properties for understanding health and disease in the body. The priority given to them by Galen is demonstrated by the opening lines of his *On Mixtures*:

> Animal bodies are a mixture of hot, cold, wet and dry; and these qualities are not mixed equally in each case.[2]

This provides Galen with a model for how health and disease can be explained on the basis of what can be easily and distinctly perceived by touch. In his system, hot, cold, wet and dry are classified as different types of interaction between physical entities. This means that in reality, they are contained within physical substances. However, this is something that Galen believes has been misunderstood by some physicians and philosophers.[3] Therefore, when Galen

---

1   Klibansky, Panofsky and Saxl, 1964: 10; Porter, 2003: 26; Hankinson, 2008: 219; Jouanna, 2006: 117–119 and 2012a: 229–230.

2   Ὅτι μὲν ἐκ θερμοῦ καὶ ψυχροῦ καὶ ξηροῦ καὶ ὑγροῦ τὰ τῶν ζῴων σώματα κέκραται καὶ ὡς οὐκ ἴση πάντων ἐστὶν ἐν τῇ κράσει μοῖρα. *Temp.* I.1 (I 509,1–3 K), translation by Singer.

3   For more information on Galen's mis-attribution of element theory to Hippocrates and his

talks about the four qualities existing within the most fundamental substances in the universe, he is referring to the cosmic elements fire, air, earth and water. This is the most basic level of matter, but when it comes to the human body (and other sanguineous animal bodies), the most basic substances within the 'proximate elements' of the body are the four humours: blood, phlegm, yellow bile and black bile. For example, in *On the Doctrines of Hippocrates and Plato*, Galen argues that Hippocrates was the first to demonstrate the true nature of substance in the body, based on the qualities, elements and humours. In this system, both the four cosmic elements and the four humours are made up of pairings of the different qualities. For Galen, both Plato and Aristotle followed Hippocrates and agreed with this model. Galen tells us that since he has discussed Hippocrates' view of the elements in great detail in *On the Elements According to Hippocrates*, and he is not in the habit of repeating himself, he will only quote the passages from Plato's writing in *On the Doctrines of Hippocrates and Plato*, where it shows agreement with Hippocrates' view of the elements. Here he is choosing to quote from Plato's *Timaeus* and wants to persuade his reader that this material is consistent with the writing of Hippocrates, such as in *On the Nature of Man*. He avoids a side by side comparison with quoted parts of this Hippocratic treatise by telling his reader to consult his other work, *On the Elements According to Hippocrates* for the material that confirms this agreement between Plato and Hippocrates on the elements.[4]

Galen regards *On the Nature of Man* as the main treatise for information on Hippocrates' work on the four humours and their relation to the four qualities, elements and the seasons of the year. For example, we find the following passage in this treatise, where each humour is associated with the qualities that predominate in each of the four seasons:

> It is chiefly in spring and summer that men are attacked by dysenteries, and by haemorrhage from the nose, and they are then hottest and red. And in summer blood is still strong, and bile rises in the body and extends until autumn. In autumn blood becomes small in quantity, as autumn is opposed to its nature, while bile prevails in the body during the summer season and during autumn. You may learn this truth from the following

---

dependence on Aristotelian natural philosophy, see Hankinson, 2008: 210–224; Kupreeva, 2014: 153–196.

4　For example, see Galen's explanation in *Hipp. Elem.* (10.1–3, CMG V 1,2, pp. 138,15–140,2 De Lacy (I 492,1–493,1 K)) for the importance of the four humours in sanguineous animals, and his argument for the general agreement between Plato and Hippocrates on the 'elements' of the body in *PHP* (VIII.2.12–4.35, CMG V 4,1,2, p. 492,22–506,3 De Lacy (V 664,8–679,16 K)).

facts. During this season men vomit bile without an emetic, and when they take purges the discharges are most bilious. It is plain too from fevers and from the complexions of men. But in summer phlegm is at its weakest. For the season is opposed to its nature, being dry and warm. But in autumn blood becomes least in man, for autumn is dry and begins from this point to chill him. It is black bile which in autumn is greatest and strongest.[5]

In Galen's *Commentary on On the Nature of Man*, when he reaches this part of the Hippocratic text, he reiterates the sections of this passage concerning the comparison of black bile with the qualities and one of the seasons of the year, as he says that 'black bile is dry and cold like autumn' (μέλαινα ... ξηρά καὶ ψυχρά, καθάπερ καὶ αὐτὸ τὸ φθινόπωρον). In an earlier section of this commentary, Galen refers to the qualities as one of the primary methods of distinguishing between the four humours.[6] We find this too in Galen's *On the Natural Faculties*, where he asks: 'is there none which is virtually cold and dry? ... No, the black bile is such a humour, ... mainly in the fall of the year, ...'[7] Similarly in *On the Doctrines of Hippocrates and Plato*: 'black [bile] is cold and dry' (ψυχρὰ δὲ ἡ μέλαινα καὶ ξηρά).[8] Whereas, in *On Mixtures*, we are told that the illness called melan-

---

5 οἱ ἄνθρωποι τοῦ ἦρος καὶ τοῦ θέρεος μάλιστα ὑπό τε τῶν δυσεντεριῶν ἁλίσκονται, καὶ ἐκ τῶν ῥινῶν τὸ αἷμα ῥεῖ αὐτοῖσι, καὶ θερμότατοί εἰσι καὶ ἐρυθροί· τοῦ δὲ θέρεος τό τε αἷμα ἰσχύει ἔτι, καὶ ἡ χολὴ αἴρεται ἐν τῷ σώματι καὶ παρατείνει ἐς τὸ φθινόπωρον· ἐν δὲ τῷ φθινοπώρῳ τὸ μὲν αἷμα ὀλίγον γίνεται, ἐναντίον γὰρ αὐτοῦ τὸ φθινόπωρον τῇ φύσει ἐστί· ἡ δὲ χολὴ τὴν θερείην κατέχει τὸ σῶμα καὶ τὸ φθινόπωρον. γνοίης δ' ἂν τοῖσδε· οἱ ἄνθρωποι αὐτόματοι ταύτην τὴν ὥρην χολὴν ἐμέουσι, καὶ ἐν τῇσι φαρμακοποσίῃσι χολωδέστατα καθαίρονται, δῆλον δὲ καὶ τοῖσι πυρετοῖσι καὶ τοῖσι χρώμασι τῶν ἀνθρώπων. τὸ δὲ φλέγμα τῆς θερείης ἀσθενέστατόν ἐστιν αὐτὸ ἑωυτοῦ· ἐναντίη γὰρ αὐτοῦ τῇ φύσει ἐστὶν ἡ ὥρη, ξηρή τε ἐοῦσα καὶ θερμή. τὸ δὲ αἷμα τοῦ φθινοπώρου ἐλάχιστον γίνεται ἐν τῷ ἀνθρώπῳ, ξηρόν τε γάρ ἐστι τὸ φθινόπωρον καὶ ψύχειν ἤδη ἄρχεται τὸν ἄνθρωπον· ἡ δὲ μέλαινα χολὴ τοῦ φθινοπώρου πλείστη τε καὶ ἰσχυροτάτη ἐστίν. *Nat. Hom.* 7, CMG I 1,3, pp. 182,19–184,14 Jouanna (VI 48,3–17 L), translation by Jones.

6 *HNH*, I.41; I.26, CMG V 9,1, pp. 51,31–32; 35,9–24 Mewaldt (XV 98,14–16; 65,3–66,5 K).

7 οὐδείς δ' ἐστὶ ψυχρὸς καὶ ξηρὸς τὴν δύναμιν ... καὶ μὴν ἥ γε μέλαινα χολὴ τοιοῦτός ἐστι χυμός ... ἐν φθινοπώρῳ μάλιστα ... *Nat. Fac.* II.9 (II 130,18–131,5 K), translation by Brock. See Siegel, 1968: 238.

8 *PHP*, VIII.4.21, CMG V 4,1,2, p. 502,22–25 De Lacy (V 676,14–19 K). Black bile is also described on the basis of the cold and dry qualities in *Morb. Diff.* (XII.2 (VI 875,9 K)) and *Caus. Morb.* (VI.3 (VII 21,17–18 K)). In *PHP* (VIII.6.1–15, CMG V 4,1,2, pp. 512,25–516,6 De Lacy (V 689,1–692,12 K)), Galen provides a more comprehensive account of all four humours, their respective qualities and the influence of the seasons on the humours. This passage is also fully quoted in Galen's *Hipp. Epid.* (II, CMG V 10,1 pp. 4,13–5,25 Pfaff). In *Temp.* (II.3; III.4 (I 603,8–14; 673,11–674,1 K)), Galen also refers to this passage when he writes about the qualities of cold and wet in phlegm. See Anastassiou and Irmer, 1997, volume II.2, pp. 277–279; II.1, pp. 363–364.

choly is cold and dry (ἢ ψυχρὸν καὶ ξηρὸν ὡς τὴν μελαγχολίαν), although this is
not a direct statement about black bile itself, it is related to an illness which
is produced by this humour.[9] This shows that the association between black
bile, autumn and the cold and dry qualities is important in Galen's theory of
this humour and that in writing about black bile in this way he is following the
ideas contained in the Hippocratic *On the Nature of Man*. This is also part of
Galen's doxographical strategy, as we find that he not only names Hippocrates
as the first to have identified this type of characterisation and association for
the four humours, but also claims that this model of the humours, based on the
pairings of the four qualities, was adopted and continued by some of the most
prominent physicians and philosophers after Hippocrates.[10]

However, Galen goes beyond what is contained in the Hippocratic *On the
Nature of Man* in his description of black bile. For example, in his commentary
on this treatise, black bile is described as being 'earth-like' (γεώδης).[11] There is
a similar statement comparing black bile to the 'cosmic element' earth in *On
the Doctrines of Hippocrates and Plato*. In this treatise Galen quotes directly
from Plato's *Timaeus* for the information regarding his discussion of the four
elements, fire, air, water and earth, but he does not provide the equivalent quotations from Hippocrates' writing that makes this comparison between black
bile and the element 'earth'. Galen cannot provide this material because there is
no clear statement in any of the works in the extant Hippocratic Corpus for this
type of association.[12] Therefore, Galen must use the similarity of the pairing of
the qualities to make this connection, and then report that Hippocrates had
made such a comparison himself.[13] This brings the seasonal characterisation
Galen has taken from *On the Nature of Man* into alignment with the theories of
the elements produced by Plato and Aristotle. This is typical of Galen's strategy
of presenting his theory as being in agreement with what he considers to be the
best medical and philosophical authorities of the past. The clear hierarchical
association between the qualities, cosmic elements and humours is important
in Galen's biological model, as it connects the human body to all the substances
in the universe by the pairing of the four qualities, hot, cold, dry and wet, in each

---

9   *Temp.* I.3 (I 522,7–8 K).

10 In *Nat. Fac.* (II.8 (II 110,12–111,10 K)), Galen lists Hippocrates with Diocles, Praxagoras, and
    Philistion, along with Plato, Aristotle and Theophrastus as the physicians and philoso-
    phers who postulated a medical system with the four qualities as its basis and the associ-
    ation with the four humours. See chapter 1, section 2 above.

11 *HNH*, I.40, CMG V 9,1, p. 50,23–25 Mewaldt (XV 96,8–10 K).

12 The only use of the term, γεώδης, is in *Diseases IV* (XXIV (55 L) (VII 600,14–20 L)), which
    refers to milk that is earthy and phlegmatic, but this does not refer to black bile.

13 *PHP*, VIII.4.21, CMG V 4,1,2, p. 502,24 De Lacy (V 676,17–18 K).

of the four cosmic elements and humours. This is why it is necessary for Galen to ignore the fact that there is no explicit association of black bile with the cosmic element 'earth' in the Hippocratic writings because what matters here is that Hippocrates and Plato are shown to be in agreement. He relies on the fact that black bile is associated with 'cold and dry' in the Hippocratic Corpus and that the elemental earth is also described in terms of these two qualities in Plato's writing. Galen is not concerned about whether the Hippocratic treatises contain direct statements about the association between black bile and the elemental earth. Instead, he reports this information, as what Hippocrates would have said if he was explicitly asked to make this connection. For Galen, it is important that there is consistency between his 'best physicians and philosophers' on the qualities, elements and humours, as this is a stronger defence against the types of rival theories based on discrete particles and atoms, which he wants to refute.

The elemental qualities are not the only way that black bile can be described as being distinct from other substances. There are a number of other key characteristics and properties that can be used to define black bile. The following passage from the Hippocratic *On the Nature of Man* provides some useful information on the way that black bile can be characterised in relation to the other three humours:

> I say they are blood, phlegm, yellow bile and black bile. First I say that the names of these according to convention are separated, and that none of them has the same name as the others; furthermore, that according to nature their essential forms are separated, phlegm being quite unlike blood, blood being quite unlike bile, bile being quite unlike phlegm. How could they be like one another, when their colours appear not alike to the sight nor does their touch seem alike to the hand? For they are not equally warm, nor cold, nor dry, nor moist. Since then they are so different from one another in essential form and in power, they cannot be one, if fire and water are not one. From the following evidence you may know that they are not all one, but that each of them has its own power and its own nature.[14]

---

14 φημὶ δὴ εἶναι αἷμα καὶ φλέγμα καὶ χολὴν ξανθὴν καὶ μέλαιναν. καὶ τούτων πρῶτον μὲν κατὰ νόμον τὰ ὀνόματα διωρίσθαι φημὶ καὶ οὐδενὶ αὐτῶν τὸ αὐτὸ ὄνομα εἶναι, ἔπειτα κατὰ φύσιν τὰς ἰδέας κεχωρίσθαι, καὶ οὔτε τὸ φλέγμα οὐδὲν ἐοικέναι τῷ αἵματι, οὔτε τὸ αἷμα τῇ χολῇ, οὔτε τὴν χολὴν τῷ φλέγματι. πῶς γὰρ ἂν ἐοικότα ταῦτα εἴη ἀλλήλοισιν, ὧν οὔτε τὰ χρώματα ὅμοια φαίνεται προσορώμενα, οὔτε τῇ χειρὶ ψαύοντι ὅμοια δοκεῖ εἶναι; οὔτε γὰρ θερμὰ ὁμοίως ἐστίν, οὔτε ψυχρά, οὔτε ξηρά, οὔτε ὑγρά. ἀνάγκη τοίνυν, ὅτε τοσοῦτον διήλλακται ἀλλήλων τὴν ἰδέην τε καὶ

This passage refers to the main differences between the four humours on the basis of their physical and qualitative properties. The first example uses a basic characterisation of colour.[15] In the naming of the four humours, as we see from the passage above, the two types of bile are distinguished by colour; yellow and black. This difference in colour can be used for all four humours to determine various types of disease. We find that Galen writes about the importance of the different colours of the humours, as he tells us that the spit of people suffering from pleurisy is often red or yellow in colour, indicating a predominance of blood or yellow bile in the body.[16] In *On the Doctrines of Hippocrates and Plato*, Galen refers to what he calls Hippocrates' method of diagnosing diseases in the body from the colour of the tongue, which indicates the predominance of each of the four humours, blood, phlegm, yellow bile and black bile, from the tongue changing to the colour of red, white, yellow and black, respectively. Here, Galen is referring to a passage from the Hippocratic *Epidemics VI*.[17] More information on Galen's interpretation of this passage can be found in his *Commentary on Epidemics*, where he tells us that the appearance of a black tongue is an indication of the presence of too much black bile in the body.[18] When Galen refers to the red, white, yellow and black colour of the tongue, he is talking about an association with the 'ideal' colours of the four humours. In many cases there will be variations in colour due to different factors, such as consistency and mixture with other substances.[19] In *On Black Bile*, Galen explains that blood can be redder (ἐρυθρότερος) from the veins, but is more yellow (ξανθότερος) from the arteries. Yellow bile can often seem to be a pale yellow (ὠχρός) colour or even like the colour of raw egg-yolk (λεκιθώδης).[20] When it comes to black bile, a black tongue can be an indication that this humour has become more dominant in the body, which can lead to certain types of illness. However, Galen is

---

τὴν δύναμιν, μὴ ἓν αὐτὰ εἶναι, εἴπερ μὴ πῦρ τε καὶ ὕδωρ ἕν ἐστιν. γνοίης δ' ἂν τοῖσδε, ὅτι οὐχ ἓν ταῦτα πάντα ἐστίν, ἀλλ' ἕκαστον αὐτῶν ἔχει δύναμίν τε καὶ φύσιν τὴν ἑωυτοῦ· *Nat. Hom.* 6, CMG I 1,3, pp. 174,12–176,11 Jouanna (VI 40,16–42,10 L), adapted from a translation by Jones.

15   Bradley, 2009: 128–129 and 131–133. For example, the first century CE physician Celsus (*Medicina*, II.4.7) writes that green or black vomit is a bad sign. When it comes to urine, red means there is a problem, but if it is 'white like flower petals' then this is even worse.

16   *CAM*, 14.18–19, CMG V 1,3, p. 102,15–24 Fortuna (I 278,2–14 K). See Bradley, 2009: 134.

17   *PHP*, VIII.5.10–13, CMG V 4,1,2, p. 506,30–508,4 De Lacy (V 681,15–682,12 K); *Epid. VI* (V.8 (V 318,5–8 L)). See Siegel, 1968: 279; Anastassiou and Irmer, 1997, volume II.2 p. 219.

18   *Hipp. Epid.* VI.I.2; VI.V.16; VI.VI.3, CMG V 10,2,2 pp. 10,5–8; 296,19–23; 328,13–17 (XVIIa 805,15–806,1; XVIIb 277,13–278,2; 322,6–10 K). See Anastassiou and Irmer, 1997, volume II.1 p. 263.

19   In *PHP* (VIII.5.17–20, CMG V 4,1,2 p. 508,14–28 De Lacy (V 683,7–684,9 K)), Galen quotes a passage from Plato's *Timaeus* (83a–c), where bile is described using different colours relating to its structure or its mixture with other humours.

20   *At. Bil.* 2, CMG V 4,1,1, pp. 72,10–12; 73,23–74,4 De Boer (V 106,6–9; 109,3–18 K).

concerned that some physicians may make an incorrect diagnosis or prognosis of a disease based purely on the observation of 'black substances' in material secreted from the body. Observation of colour alone is not reliable enough to make a precise identification of black bile, as there are natural variations in the colours of the humours caused by consistency and mixture. In addition, there are many similar substances that are black, which could be mistaken for black bile. Fortunately, there are other characteristics that can be used to identify this humour.

In the passage from *On the Nature of Man* quoted above (page 64), we find 'that according to nature their essential forms are separated, phlegm being quite unlike blood, blood being quite unlike bile, bile being quite unlike phlegm'. This indicates that form (ἰδέη) is an important determinant for the identification of a humour. We have already seen (see pages 63–64 above) that Galen associates black bile with the elemental 'earth' and so its density and thickness come from both its cold and dry qualities and its earth-like nature. For example, in Galen's *Commentary on On the Nature of Man*, black bile can be identified using this parameter of thickness:

> Black bile, in turn, is always thicker than the pale or yellow bile. And in black bile, the difference between the greater thickness and the lesser is not slight, just as is the case with blood.[21]

Galen uses the word 'thick' (παχύς) to describe the relative density of three of the humours. In addition, we find the same term being used by him in *On the Elements According to Hippocrates*, *On Mixtures*, and *On Black Bile* to describe black bile as being a thick substance.[22] The relatively thick nature of black bile is something that Galen uses to describe this humour so that it may be identified correctly. In this way, he is emphasising the importance of certain characteristics that can be used to determine the possibility of whether a particular black substance may be identified as being the black bile humour or not. One point to note is that Galen is using the term παχύς to express the thickness of black bile in his *Commentary on On the Nature of Man*, even though this term is not actually used to describe black bile in the Hippocratic *On the Nature of*

---

21   ἥ τ' αὖ μέλαινα διὰ παντός ἐστι παχυτέρα τῆς ὠχρᾶς τε καὶ ξανθῆς, οὐκ ὀλίγον δὲ οὐδὲ κατὰ ταύ-
       την ἐστὶ τὸ μᾶλλόν τε καὶ ἧττον, ὥσπερ γε καὶ κατὰ τὸ αἷμα· ΗΝΗ, 1.26, CMG V 9,1, p. 36,3–5
       Mewaldt (xv 66,13–16 κ), translation by Lewis.
22   For example, in *Hipp. Elem.* 13.23, CMG V 4,1, p. 154,8–10 (1 506,5–7 κ); *Temp.* 11.3 (1 603,9–11
       κ); *At. Bil.* 3, CMG V 4,1,1, pp. 74,26–75,1 De Boer (V 111,9–12 κ).

Man, or any of the other extant texts in the Hippocratic Corpus.[23] However, we can see that the notion of black bile as a thick substance is found in the Hippocratic Corpus when there is a reference to its relative viscosity (see below). This is an example of Galen's choice of terminology that does not necessarily coincide with what is found in the Hippocratic Corpus, but is compatible with the physical description of black bile in some of the Hippocratic treatises.

The use of παχύς is not the only way to describe the structural density of black bile. Other qualities also indicate black bile's relative thickness. We have seen that black bile is characterised as a cold and dry humour. When it comes to the 'cold' quality, both yellow bile and blood are hotter humours than black bile and from everyday experience we find that hot fluids tend to flow more freely than cold ones. If we apply the same reasoning to the 'dry' quality, we would expect a dry substance like black bile to flow less freely than 'moist' blood. Both black bile and yellow bile are classified as 'dry', but black bile, being colder, will be more viscous. Therefore on the basis of the qualities of cold and dry, we would expect black bile to be a 'thicker' substance than yellow bile and blood. But what about the relative thickness of black bile compared to phlegm, which is characterised as a cold and moist humour?

If we investigate *On Mixtures*, we find that Galen regards black bile as being colder and thicker than blood, but phlegm is the coldest and wettest of all the four humours. Galen also refers to phlegm as a particularly sticky substance, but he does not provide any comparative information between phlegm and the other humours in this context.[24] Further to this, there are two places in *On Black Bile* where viscosity is used, but these are more general cases referring to the cause of disease by substances that are viscous, which includes black bile. But there is no separate statement to say that black bile is the 'stickiest' of the four humours.[25] In addition to these examples, in *On the Therapeutic Method* Galen describes phlegm as being thicker (παχύτερον) and stickier (γλί-σχρον) than yellow bile, and like black bile, phlegm is more difficult to evacuate from the body.[26] Here we find that Galen is following the same characterisation of the structural form of the humours, which is found in the quoted passage

---

23 There is a reference in the Hippocratic *Aer.* (X (II 50,10–14 L)) to a thick residue when the humid and watery part of bile is dried up. But the author of this text does not refer explicitly to this residue as 'black bile'.

24 μέλαινα γὰρ χολὴ τῶν ἐν τῷ σώματι ἐνεόντων χυμῶν γλισχρότατον, καὶ τὰς ἕδρας χρονιωτά-τας ποιεῖται. *Temp.* II.3 (I 603,10–11 K). There are references to phlegm being a particularly sticky substance in *Temp.* (III.4 (I 673,16–674,1 K)).

25 *At. Bil.* 5; 7, CMG V 4,1,1, pp. 81,27–28; 86,25–28 De Boer (V 125,8–10; 134,12–16 K).

26 *MM*, XIV.16 (X 1010,2–5 K).

from *On the Nature of Man*.[27] Therefore, when it comes to structural consistency, black bile is considered by Galen as a thick and sticky humour, which is difficult to remove from the body. This suggests that Galen does not think that this issue of which humour is the 'stickiest' is important enough to require detailed analysis and explanation of the relevant parts of the Hippocratic writings. We are therefore left at this point with the only clear information being that black bile is thicker, stickier and colder than blood and yellow bile, but drier and less cold than phlegm. It is the case that Galen draws upon the characterisation of black bile in *On the Nature of Man*, describing it as a cold, dry substance, which is the thickest and most viscous of the four humours. The inertia of black bile in the body, due to its sticky nature, will become important because its physical effect on the body can cause specific diseases, which I will discuss later.[28]

2   Physical Descriptions of Black Bile

We have seen already that Galen, in general, has been consistent with the Hippocratic *On the Nature of Man* to describe black bile as being a black, cold, dry, thick and sticky substance. Galen believed that it was important to provide such detailed information, so that physicians would be able to identify the presence of black bile in the waste products evacuated from the body during an illness. For example, we find the following description in *On the Natural Faculties*:

> Next, two residues produced by way of the change of this, the one being more light and air-like and the other being more heavy and earth-like; of these the one, as I understand, they call the flower and the other the lees. Of these you will not be wrong comparing yellow bile with the [former] one of these two, black bile with the [latter] one of these two, ...[29]

In this passage, black bile is compared to the lees, which are described as 'heavy and earth-like'. This is similar to the characterisation that we saw earlier, when

---

27   *Nat. Hom.* 7; 15, CMG I 1,3, pp. 182,6–9; 204,12–14 Jouanna (VI 46,13–14; 68,6–8 L).
28   See chapter 7 below.
29   ἔπειτα κατὰ τὴν αὐτοῦ μεταβολὴν δύο γεννώμενα περιττώματα τὸ μὲν κουφότερόν τε καὶ ἀερωδέ-
      στερον, τὸ δὲ βαρύτερόν τε καὶ γεωδέστερον, ὧν τὸ μὲν ἄνθος, οἶμαι, τὸ δὲ τρύγα καλοῦσι. τούτων
      τῷ μὲν ἑτέρῳ τὴν ξανθὴν χολήν, τῷ δ' ἑτέρῳ τὴν μέλαιναν εἰκάζων οὐκ ἂν ἁμάρτοις, ... *Nat. Fac.*
      II.9 (II 135,6–11 K), adapted from a translation by Brock.

black bile was associated with the elemental 'earth' (see pages 63–64 above). However, I want to focus on the description of black bile as being like 'lees' (τρύξ). In the medical texts, we find that this term τρύξ is most commonly used for the lees of wine, which are the particles of yeast or other solid matter found in some types of wine. Galen includes this description in other treatises, such as *On Black Bile* where he uses both terms 'melancholic humour' (μελαγχολι-κὸς χυμός) and 'black bile' (μέλαινα χολή) when he describes black bile as being like the 'lees in wine' (ἐν οἴνῳ ἡ τρύξ).[30] He also uses a more direct characterisation of black bile relative to blood when he refers to μέλαινα χολή as the 'lees of blood' (τρύγα τοῦ αἵματος), which we can find in *On Crises* and in his *Commentary on Aphorisms*.[31] Therefore, Galen is reinforcing his description of black bile by saying that this humour should be considered as being the lees of blood. In other words when you look at composite blood, the part that is heavy, which resembles the lees, is in fact black bile.

We can see that Galen is utilising a well-known and observable substance, in this case 'lees' (τρύξ), for his description of a thick black substance, found in certain fluids, which he identifies as black bile. If we investigate the Hippocratic Corpus, we find a similar description in *On Diseases II*. In this case, some of the substances found in vomit are called dark like lees (οἷον τρύγα), which sometimes looks like blood (τοτὲ δὲ αἱματῶδες), and sometimes like second-wine (τοτὲ δὲ οἷον οἶνον τὸν δεύτερον).[32] Further to this, there are a couple of examples of the use of the term τρύξ in the Hippocratic *Epidemics V* and *Epidemics VII*. For example, we are told that a certain Eutychides had a choleric illness ending with him vomiting material that contained lees.[33] We have seen earlier that Galen had rejected the general content of *On Diseases II*, *Epidemics V* and *VII* as inauthentic.[34] However, it is possible that Galen may have drawn upon the passage from *On Diseases II* for his characterisation of black bile, as he may be referring to this passage in his *Glossary of Hippocratic Terms*.[35] The reason why Galen is writing about the appearance of black bile in this way is that it is useful to doctors, as they will be familiar with the appearance of lees in wine and therefore they will be able to look for a similar substance in the different types of waste fluids secreted from the body.

---

30 *At. Bil.* 6, CMG V 4,1,1, p. 83,13 De Boer (V 127,15–16 K). See also *At. Bil.* 3; 7, (pp. 75,8–12; 87,8–10 (V 112,2–8; 135,11–12 K)).

31 *Cris.* II.12 (IX 694,6–10 K); *Hipp. Aph.* IV.21 (XVIIb 682,1 K).

32 *Morb. II*, 73,1 (VII 110,14–15 L).

33 *Epid. V*, 1,79,6 (V 248,22 L); *Epid. VII*, 1,67,6 (V 430,15–16 L).

34 See chapter 2, section 3 above.

35 I will be discussing Galen's use of this passage from *On Diseases II* in more detail later, see chapter 5, section 1 below.

The description of black bile as a solid within other fluids is emphasised by Galen in another of his works. In *On Mixtures*, we find the following description being applied to black bile:

> Of humours the most useful and particular is blood. Black bile is a kind of sediment and mud of this [blood]; it is therefore colder and thicker than blood.[36]

This is a distinctive characterisation of black bile relative to blood and is not found applied to the other two humours, phlegm and yellow bile in any of Galen's extant writing. This is understandable in the case of yellow bile, since this humour is considered to be hot and thin and therefore would not form a heavy precipitate like this. However, as we have seen earlier, phlegm is described as being a viscous substance (see pages 67–68 above), so there is the possibility that it could form white sediment in blood. But Galen does not describe the physical appearance of phlegm in this way, and so it seems that sediment and mud found in blood is reserved for black bile.[37] The use of sediment (ὑπόστασις) to characterise black bile in blood is only found explicitly like this in *On Mixtures*. If we look in the Hippocratic Corpus for ὑπόστασις, we find that there are no similar direct statements that black bile is a type of sediment of blood in this way. Instead, there are some passages where sediment is observed in the evacuated waste from the body. For example, the authors of *Epidemics I* and *III* refer to patients with fever who have black sediment (ὑπόστασις) in their urine and faeces respectively.[38] Another example is found in *Koan Prognoses*, where the presence of black ὑπόστασις in urine is a mortal sign.[39] The authors of these passages use sediment as a description of the physical material in waste matter, but this is not the same as the characterisation of black bile as sediment in blood, which we have seen in Galen's *On Mixtures*. We know that Galen acknowledged *Epidemics I* and *III* as being some of the best works written by Hippocrates and he also believed that parts of *Koan Prognoses* were of a standard consistent with a genuine Hippocratic work.[40] However,

---

36 Τῶν δὲ χυμῶν ὁ μὲν χρηστότατός τε καὶ οἰκειότατός ἐστι τὸ αἷμα. τούτου δ' οἷον ὑπόστασίς τις καὶ ἰλὺς ἡ μέλαινα χολή· ταῦτ' ἄρα καὶ ψυχροτέρα τ' ἐστὶ καὶ παχυτέρα τοῦ αἵματος· *Temp*. II.3 (I 603,7–10 K), adapted from a translation by Singer.

37 In fact, we find that in *At. Bil.* (2, CMG V 4,1,1, p. 73,1–2 De Boer (V 107,12–13 K)), Galen describes the appearance of phlegm in blood as the opposite of sediment, as he says that phlegm can sometimes be seen to float on the surface of blood.

38 *Epid. I*, Case II (II 684,16–17 L); *Epid. III*, Case III (III 40,12–13 L).

39 *Coac*. 569 and 570 (V 714,15–16 and 716,3–4 L).

40 See chapter 2, section 3 above.

although there are no quotations or references to any of these examples of black sediment in the majority of the extant works by Galen, he does comment on the passages from *Epidemics I* and *III* in his *Commentary on Epidemics*. In both cases of the black sediment found in waste material from the body, Galen warns that this is a bad sign of unconcocted and potentially destructive material in the body. It is significant that Galen does not refer to this black sediment as indicating the presence of harmful 'black bile' or 'melancholic humour' in the body when he interprets these passages. Instead, he refers to a more general type of harmful substance in the body. This might indicate that Galen does not want this substance to be identified as black bile for the purposes of diagnosis and prognosis at this specific point in the text.[41] If we investigate some of the Aristotelian sources, we find in the pseudo-Aristotelian *Problemata* that there is a comparison between 'black bile' (μέλαινα χολή) and the build-up of a type of 'sediment' (ὑπόστασις) in the body when a person is suffering from quartan fever. But, again we do not find black bile being characterised as sediment in blood.[42] Therefore, there is precedence for this term ὑπόστασις being used to describe substances in evacuated material from the body that indicate that there is something potentially harmful in the body. But Galen's use of ὑπόστασις is different from these Hippocratic and Aristotelian sources, as he characterises black bile as a type of sediment in blood. This is something that Galen believes is useful for the identification of black bile.

In addition to ὑπόστασις, we can see in the passage from *On Mixtures* (see page 70 above) that Galen also describes black bile as 'mud' (ἰλύς) in blood. The use of ἰλύς might indicate a more solid kind of matter in relation to other substances that are present, in this case blood. We also find this characterisation in *On Black Bile*, where again Galen refers to black bile as being like ἰλύς in blood. But, in contrast to the more direct statement in *On Mixtures*, this is a more general statement about the need to remove impurities from the blood.[43] We also find ἰλύς in *On the Elements According to Hippocrates*, but this time, Galen is not actually referring to black bile.[44] However, in addition to what we have found in *On Mixtures* and *On Black Bile*, the description of black bile as

---

41   *Hipp. Epid.* I.III.19, CMG V 10,1, p. 133,5–25 Wenkebach (XVIIa 265,4–266,6 K); III.I.25, CMG V 10,2,1, p. 52,5–8 Wenkebach (XVIIa 567,13–568,2 K).

42   Pseudo-Aristotle, *Pr.* I.19, 861b19–21. I will be discussing black bile as the cause of quartan fever in more detail later, see chapter 7, section 2 below.

43   *At. Bil.* 7, CMG V 4,1,1, p. 87,8–10 De Boer (V 135,10–13 K).

44   Galen uses both ἰλύς and τρύξ in his analogy between the composite form of blood and milk in *Hipp. Elem.* (11.11, CMG V 1,2, p. 142,23–25 De Lacy (I 496,6–10 K)), but he does not mention here that these terms can also be applied to black bile.

being like mud in its appearance is quite common in Galen's writing. For example, in *On the Therapeutic Method, On the Power of Cleansing Drugs* and *On the Composition of Drugs According to Places*, thick blood that resembles mud is associated with black bile.[45] This shows that Galen was characterising black bile as a more solid substance than the other three humours and that black bile can be observed as a type of black matter, which appears as a muddy substance in blood. An attempt to trace this form of black bile in the Hippocratic Corpus does not yield any explicit reference to black bile being characterised as 'the mud of blood' in this way.[46] However, if we investigate Aristotelian works, although there are no references to black bile as appearing like mud, there is a passage in *Parts of Animals* that discusses the effect of 'the mud of dark wine' (ἡ ἰλὺς τοῦ μέλανος οἴνου) on the colour of the 'residue discharges' (περιττώματα) from the stomach.[47] We find that from an overall Aristotelian perspective there may be some close association between the 'mud of dark wine' and 'black bile'. For instance, there is Aristotle's characterisation of black bile as a residue and a comparison between the cause of melancholy with the effect of dark wine to produce inebriation in the pseudo-Aristotelian *Problemata*.[48] Potentially, this could have influenced Galen's writing on this type of physical description of black bile.

We are now a long way from the characterisation of black bile purely on the basis of the qualities 'cold and dry' and we have seen that Galen emphasises the importance of a physical description of black bile. Therefore, Galen has gone beyond the simple cold, dry and sticky substance found in the Hippocratic *On the Nature of Man* to create a broader description of black bile, which is compared to common organic substances, such as 'lees' (τρύξ), 'sediment' (ὑπόστασις) and 'mud' (ἰλύς). These are the types of characterisation of black bile or black substances, which are found in a range of sources beyond the ideas contained in *On the Nature of Man*. We have found these descriptions in other texts from the Hippocratic Corpus, such as *On Diseases II* and some of the

---

45   *MM*, XIII.16 (X 916,13–15 K); *Purg. Med. Fac.* III (XI 335,13–17 K); *Comp. Med. Loc.* VIII.6 (XIII 197,3–5 K).

46   We find ἰλύς being used in the Hippocratic *Aer.* (IX (II 38,7–8 L)) to explain the presence of sediment of mud, which appears in the vessels of the body from the drinking of certain types of water. In the Hippocratic *Epid. VII* (XI (V 384,14–16 L)), this word is used to describe the muddy appearance of faecal matter, which is similar to its use in *Coac.* (456; 512; 567; 571 (V 686,10–12; 702,13–17; 712,19–714,7; 716,5–16 L)). In *Mul. I* (66,25–27 (VIII 138,1–2 L)), there is reference to the dregs of an ointment. However, none of these examples are referring to black bile or blood.

47   Aristotle, *PA*, III.3, 664b16–17.

48   Aristotle, *HA*, III.2, 511b1–11; Pseudo-Aristotle, *Pr.* XXX.1, 953a33–954a7.

books from the *Epidemics*. There are also some similar descriptions used as a comparison to black bile in some Aristotelian works. This shows that empirical information to form a consistent and useful description of black bile was more important to Galen than just basing the characterisation of black bile on the elemental qualities and its structural form of being thick and sticky that we find in *On the Nature of Man*. In this way *On the Nature of Man* is just one source out of many that he can draw upon from the rest of the Hippocratic writings, and other material from some of the physicians and philosophers who wrote about medicine in the several centuries between the writing of the Hippocratic works and the second century CE. Galen's aim is to present the physical description of black bile in a way that satisfies both the theoretical information, from the model of paired qualities which we find in texts like *On the Nature of Man*, and the kind of empirical information that is found in other texts from the Hippocratic Corpus, such as *On Diseases II*, the *Epidemics*, and also the comparative description of different substances with black bile found in Aristotelian works. All of this theoretical and empirical information is presented by Galen in his own biological model of human health and disease.

3 Summary

We have seen that it has been generally accepted that Galen's writing about the black bile humour is developed from the Hippocratic *On the Nature of Man*. What we find is that Galen presents an innate form of black bile that is essential for the health of the body as a cold and dry substance. But, Galen also uses the term 'thick' (παχύς) to describe black bile, which might be more receptive to his second century CE audience and more compatible with a wider set of sources than just the Hippocratic writings, such as in the works of Plato and Aristotle. Galen also goes beyond the ideas contained in *On the Nature of Man* when he associates black bile with the elemental 'earth'. This allows him to show in *On the Doctrines of Hippocrates and Plato* that Hippocrates and Plato are in agreement about this association, as in *On the Nature of Man* black bile is 'cold and dry' and in Plato's *Timaeus* 'earth' is also 'cold and dry'. Further to this, Galen has described the physical appearance of black bile in three different ways: 'lees' (τρύξ), 'sediment' (ὑπόστασις) and 'mud' (ἰλύς). This is extremely important for Galen, as if these types of substance are present in the evacuated waste, then the diagnosis will indicate that black bile may be the cause of the illness suffered by the patient. This is not the description of black bile that is found in the Hippocratic *On the Nature of Man*, but Galen attempts to show that this type of observation of black bile is consistent with Hippocrates' writing, which provides him with the authenticity and doxography that he requires for his arguments against rival theories. However, as we have seen, Galen does not combine all this theoretical and observational information about black bile in one treatise. Instead, he has the flexibility to use whichever characterisation of black bile is useful to him in a particular argument. I now want to investigate whether Galen is discussing the same substance, or different forms of black bile, when he defines and characterises this humour in his writing.

CHAPTER 4

Galen's Distinction of Different Types of Black Bile

There could be a potential problem for Galen, if black bile is both an essential humour for our health and the cause of some very deadly diseases. However, we shall see that he resolves this issue by postulating three main types of black bile, one that is natural and ideal, one that is natural but non-ideal and another that is unnatural with specific properties that explain how it can cause severe harm to parts of the body. This system of three different kinds of black bile is important for us to understand how Galen can incorporate a wide range of sources: Hippocratic and non-Hippocratic, medical and philosophical; to produce a theory that can account for both health and disease relating to substances that are collectively named black bile.

1   The Different Types of Black Bile in Galen's Writing

So far I have discussed Galen's characterisation of black bile as if it were a single substance, which is the way that it is presented in the Hippocratic *On the Nature of Man*. However, Galen's biological theory contains reference to different types of black bile with various properties, which explains how they function and affect the health of the body. For example, the following passage from *On Affected Parts* defines three types of substance relating to the black bile humour:

> Likewise the melancholic humour clearly shows different kinds of composition. One kind is like the sediment of blood and clearly manifests itself as quite thick, similar to the lees of wine. The other kind is much thinner in composition than that, and it appears acid to those who vomit or smell it; this also corrodes earth, it raises, ferments and stirs up bubbles like those that comes to the surface of a boiling soup. The one which I said resembles thick sediment does not produce the fermentation when it is poured out over the earth, unless it happens to have been burnt very intensely during a state of burning fever, and it only has very little share in the quality of acidity. Hence I am used to calling it melancholic humour or melancholic blood, for I think that it is not yet proper to call it black bile. For that humour is generated in some people in large quantity either as a result of their initial mixture or by a habit of eating

foods that change into this during the digestion within the blood vessels.[1]

This passage tells us that Galen differentiates between what he calls 'black bile' (μέλαινα χολή) and 'melancholic humour' (μελαγχολικός χυμός). We can see that μέλαινα χολή refers to the innate humour and this definition is consistent with Galen's use of this term in treatises such as *On the Elements According to Hippocrates* and *On the Doctrines of Hippocrates and Plato* because he is using the characterisation of black bile found in the Hippocratic *On the Nature of Man*. But, there are also two types of μελαγχολικός χυμός defined in the passage from *On Affected Parts*, one that is described as the 'sediment of blood' (τρύξ αἵματος), which is 'thick' (παχύς) like the 'lees of wine' (τρύξ οἴνου). Galen also names this as 'melancholic blood' (μελαγχολικόν αἷμα). The other type of melancholic humour is a substance that is thinner, acidic and effervesces when in contact with the ground. The use of 'acidic' here comes from the Greek word ὀξὺς, which is different from our modern concept of a chemical acid and should be thought of as the sensation of an acid, such as in the taste of vinegar.[2] This acidic melancholic humour is very important in Galen's explanation of diseases caused by black bile, which I will discuss in more detail later. If we return to the thick, sediment-like melancholic humour (or melancholic blood), we can see in the passage from *On Affected Parts* above that Galen is keen to emphasise that it is different from innate black bile (one of the four humours) and it is not correct to call it 'black bile' (μέλαινα χολή). However, we have seen above (pages 68–69) that Galen refers to μέλαινα χολή as the lees of blood in *On Crises* and in his *Commentary on Aphorisms*, and as a type of sediment in blood in *On Mixtures*. In these cases there is no indication that Galen is talking about a different type of black bile that is distinct from the innate humoral form. However, in the context of *On Affected Parts* it is important for Galen to differentiate between these two forms of black bile. This is because he is reluctant to associate the innate,

---

1 ὡσαύτως δὲ καὶ ὁ μελαγχολικὸς χυμὸς ἐν τῇ συστάσει σαφεῖς ἔχει τὰς διαφοράς, ὁ μὲν οἷον τρὺξ αἵματος, ἐναργῶς φαινόμενος ἱκανῶς παχύς, ὥσπερ ἡ τοῦ οἴνου τρύξ· ὁ δὲ πολλῷ μὲν τούτου λεπτότερος κατὰ τὴν σύστασιν, ὀξὺς δὲ καὶ τοῖς ἐμέσασιν αὐτὸν φαινόμενος καὶ τοῖς ὀσμωμένοις· οὗτος καὶ ξύει τὴν γῆν, ἐξαίρων τε καὶ ζυμῶν καὶ πομφόλυγας ἐγείρων, οἷαι τοῖς ζέουσι ζωμοῖς ἐφίστανται· ὃν δ' ἔφην ἐοικέναι παχείᾳ τρυγί, τήν τε ζύμωσιν οὐκ ἐργάζεται κατὰ τῆς γῆς ἐκχυθείς, πλὴν εἰ μὴ πάνυ σφόδρα τύχοι τότε κατοπτηθεὶς ἐν διακαεῖ πυρετῷ, καὶ ἥκιστα μετέχει ποιότητος ὀξείας, ἡνίκα καὶ καλεῖν αὐτὸν εἴωθα μελαγχολικὸν χυμὸν ἢ μελαγχολικὸν αἷμα, μέλαιναν γὰρ χολὴν οὐδέπω δικαιῶ τὸν τοιοῦτον ὀνομάζειν. γεννᾶται δ' ὁ χυμὸς οὗτος ἐνίοις πολύς, ἢ διὰ τὴν ἐξ ἀρχῆς κρᾶσιν, ἢ δι' ἔθος ἐδεσμάτων εἰς τοιοῦτον χυμὸν ἐν τῇ κατὰ τὰς φλέβας πέψει μεταβαλόντων. *Loc. Aff.* III.9 (VIII 176,15–177,12 K), translation by van der Eijk.

2 Galen, *SMT* I.39 (XI 453,14–17 K). See Siegel, 1968: 259.

fundamental μέλαινα χολή humour with the illness of melancholy directly. This is due to the sources that he has used to produce his theory of how people can suffer from a mental illness like melancholy.[3] It is important to note that Galen is able to reestablish the connection between the μέλαινα χολή and μελαγχολικός χυμός forms of black bile here, as he says that the μελαγχολικός χυμός has the potential to become μέλαινα χολή during the processing of this humour by the spleen.

There are other examples of Galen making this type of distinction between different types of substance that are related in some way to the black bile humour. For example, in the following passage from Galen's *Commentary on Aphorisms*:

> It is necessary to mention the distinctions that were made in other writings concerning black bile, since the one of them arising from yellow bile has been excessively heated, this is the one that is most difficult in all cases, and the other that comes from mud and lees, as you might say, of blood, this latter has a thicker consistency and falls short in the badness of its quality. It has been said that when we are being precise we do not call the lees of blood black bile, but rather melancholic humour. But when we are using terms loosely, we use black [bile], because it is going to become black [bile] if we do not remove it first.[4]

We can see that it is important for Galen that he makes a clear distinction between the physical properties of these two types of 'black bile', one that is described as the 'mud and lees' of blood and the other that is very harmful and is produced from the heating of yellow bile. This latter type has the same properties as the acidic type of black bile, which is referred to in the passage from *On Affected Parts* above. At the end of the passage from *Commentary on Aphorisms*, we can see that precise language is required to distinguish between μέλαινα χολή and μελαγχολικός χυμός, but Galen admits that the potential for

---

3 See chapter 7, section 1 below.

4 μεμνῆσθαι γὰρ χρὴ τῶν περὶ τῆς μελαίνης χολῆς ἐν ἄλλοις διωρισμένων, ὡς ἡ μὲν ὑπεροπτηθείσης γίνεται τῆς ξανθῆς χολῆς, ἥπερ δὴ καὶ χαλεπωτάτη παντοίως ἐστίν, ἡ δ' ἐκ τῆς τοῦ αἵματος, ὡς ἂν εἴποι τις, ἰλύος καὶ τρυγός. παχυτέρα μὲν ἐκείνη τῇ συστάσει, πολὺ δὲ ἀπολειπομένη τῷ μοχθηρῷ τῆς ποιότητος. εἴρηται δὲ καὶ ὅτι τὴν οἷον τρύγα τοῦ αἵματος ἀκριβολογούμενοι μὲν οὐδέπω μέλαιναν χολὴν ὀνομάζομεν, ἀλλὰ μελαγχολικὸν χυμόν, καταχρώμενοι δὲ τοῖς ὀνόμασι καὶ μέλαιναν ἐστιν ὅτε καλοῦμεν, ἐπειδὴ μικρὸν ὕστερον ἔσεσθαι μέλλει μέλαινα μὴ φθασάντων κενῶσαι. *Hipp. Aph.* VI.53 (XVIIIa 91,6–16 K). I would like to thank David Leith and John Wilkins for their help with the translation of this passage.

μελαγχολικός χυμός to be transformed into black bile permits the use of μέλαινα χολή. This implies that Galen is using language more loosely in texts, such as *On Crises*, *On Mixtures*, and even other sections of *Commentary on Aphorisms*, when he refers to the sediment, muddy or lees of blood substances as μέλαινα χολή rather than μελαγχολικός χυμός.

We can find a justification of this type of 'looseness' of language in a passage at the end of Galen's *On Black Bile*:

> By a process of homonymy for themselves, but not for us, they deal in subtleties about the melancholic humour, which we say is engendered in healthy people, as I always understand that it is said in contrast to black bile, which we say is created in an unnatural state because the black bile in people that are absolutely healthy is not the same as those who are in an unnatural state, but nothing prevents me from calling both melancholic humour.[5]

In this passage, Galen is drawing attention to the fact that he understands that there is a difference between black bile that is produced in someone that is healthy and in a person who is in a 'unnatural state' (παρὰ φύσιν).[6] He warns that there are some people, whom he does not name, who use μελαγχολικός χυμός as if it refers to the same type of black bile. Galen claims that he can use 'melancholic humour' for both types of black bile because he knows the important differences between them. This is particularly important when it comes to identifying them in the waste material evacuated from the body during illness, as it will affect diagnosis and prognosis.

Another example of Galen's reference to different types of black bile can be found in *On the Natural Faculties*. We find again that Galen discusses issues with the naming of such substances:

---

5   καὶ μέντοι καὶ παρὰ τὴν ὁμωνυμίαν ἑαυτούς, οὐ γὰρ ἡμᾶς γε, σοφίζονται τόν γε μελαγχολικὸν χυμόν, ὃν ἐν τοῖς ὑγιαίνουσι γεννᾶσθαί φαμεν, ἀκούοντες ἀεὶ κατὰ τῆς μελαίνης λέγεσθαι χολῆς, ἣν ἐν τῷ παρὰ φύσιν ἔχειν γεννᾶσθαί φαμεν. οὐ γὰρ ἡ αὐτὴ κατά γε τοὺς ἀκριβῶς ὑγιαίνοντάς ἐστι μέλαινα χολὴ καί τινας τῶν παρὰ φύσιν ἐχόντων, ἀμφοτέρας δὲ μελαγχολικὸν χυμὸν ὀνομάζειν οὐδὲν κωλύει. *At. Bil.* 8, CMG V 4,1,1, p. 93,22–28 De Boer (V 147,9–148,1 K), adapted from a translation by Grant. I would like to thank David Leith and John Wilkins for their help with the translation of this passage.

6   Earlier in *At. Bil.* (8, CMG V 4,1,1, p. 92,9–22 De Boer (V 144,13–145,11 K)), Galen had informed us that some people (as usual he does not name them) have denied the existence of black bile in those who have a healthy constitution and that this humour is only produced in people that have a constitution that is contrary to nature (παρὰ φύσιν).

... on the other hand, the black bile itself [becomes] much more malignant than the according to nature [black bile]; no particular name has been given to such a humour, except that some people have called it corrosive or acidic, because it also becomes acidic like vinegar and corrodes the animal's body, and the ground, if it be poured out upon it, and it produces a kind of fermentation and seething, accompanied by bubbles, an abnormal putrefaction having become added to the according to nature black humour. It seems to me also that most of the ancient physicians give the name black humour and not black bile to the according to nature portion of this humour, which is discharged from the bowel and which also frequently rises to the top [of the stomach-contents]; and they call black bile that part which, through a kind of combustion and putrefaction, has had its quality changed to acid ... Similarly with the black humour: that which does not yet produce, as I say, this seething and fermentation on the ground, is according to nature, while that which changes to such a form and faculty, is contrary to nature; it has assumed an acridity owing to the combustion caused by contrary to nature heat, and has practically become transformed into ashes. In somewhat the same way burned lees differ from unburned. The former is a warm substance, able to burn, dissolve, and destroy the flesh. The other kind, which has not yet undergone combustion, one may find the physicians employing for the same purposes that one uses the so-called potter's earth and other substances which have naturally a combined drying and chilling action.[7]

In this passage we have one type of black bile that is less harmful and is described as being 'according to nature' (κατὰ φύσιν). In contrast, another type

---

7 ... ἡ δ' αὖ μέλαινα κακοηθέστερα μὲν πολὺ καὶ αὕτη τῆς κατὰ φύσιν· ὄνομα δ' οὐδὲν ἴδιον κεῖται τῷ τοιούτῳ χυμῷ, πλὴν εἴ πού τινες ἢ ξυστικὸν ἢ ὀξῶδη κεκλήκασιν αὐτόν, ὅτι καὶ δριμὺς ὁμοίως ὄξει γίγνεται καὶ ξύει γε τὸ σῶμα τοῦ ζῴου καὶ τὴν γῆν, εἰ κατ' αὐτῆς ἐκχυθείη, καί τινα μετὰ πομφολύ-γων οἷον ζύμωσίν τε καὶ ζέσιν ἐργάζεται, σηπεδόνος ἐπικτήτου προσελθούσης ἐκείνῳ τῷ κατὰ φύσιν ἔχοντι χυμῷ τῷ μέλανι. καί μοι δοκοῦσιν οἱ πλεῖστοι τῶν παλαιῶν ἰατρῶν αὐτὸ μὲν τὸ κατὰ φύσιν ἔχον τοῦ τοιούτου χυμοῦ καὶ διαχωροῦν κάτω καὶ πολλάκις ἐπιπολάζον ἄνω μέλανα καλεῖν χυμόν, οὐ μέλαιναν χολήν, τὸ δ' ἐκ συγκαύσεώς τινος καὶ σηπεδόνος εἰς τὴν ὀξεῖαν μεθιστάμενον ποιότητα μέλαιναν ὀνομάζειν χολήν ... ὥσπερ γε καὶ τοῦ μέλανος χυμοῦ τὸ μὲν μήπω τὴν οἷον ζέσιν τε καὶ ζύμωσιν τῆς γῆς ἐργαζόμενον κατὰ φύσιν ἐστί, τὸ δ' εἰς τοιαύτην μεθιστάμενον ἰδέαν τε καὶ δύναμιν ἤδη παρὰ φύσιν, ὡς ἂν τὴν ἐκ τῆς συγκαύσεως τοῦ παρὰ φύσιν θερμοῦ προσειληφὸς δριμύτητα καὶ οἷον τέφρα τις ἤδη γεγονός. ὧδέ πως καὶ ἡ κεκαυμένη τρὺξ τῆς ἀκαύστου διήνεγκε. θερμὸν γάρ τι χρῆμα αὕτη γ' ἱκανῶς ἐστιν, ὥστε καίειν τε καὶ τήκειν καὶ διαφθείρειν τὴν σάρκα. τῇ δ' ἑτέρᾳ τῇ μήπω κεκαυμένῃ τοὺς ἰατροὺς ἔστιν εὑρεῖν χρωμένους εἰς ὅσαπερ καὶ τῇ γῇ τῇ καλουμένῃ κεραμίτιδι καὶ τοῖς ἄλλοις, ὅσα ξηραίνειν θ' ἅμα καὶ ψύχειν πέφυκεν. Nat. Fac. II.9 (II 135,16–136,11; 137,5–17 K), adapted from a translation by Brock.

of black bile is said to be very harmful to the body, as it is acidic, corrosive and effervesces when in contact with the ground.[8] Galen refers to this type of black bile as 'contrary to nature' (παρὰ φύσιν). He discusses these two descriptions based on the nomenclature used by some of the ancient physicians. So we find that the κατὰ φύσιν type was called 'black humour' (μέλας χυμός), and the παρὰ φύσιν type was named μέλαινα χολή by them.[9] Galen does not name these 'ancient physicians' at this point, but it is possible that this is the nomenclature used by Diocles to classify two different states of black bile.[10] However, we do not find this explicit distinction between two types of black bile in any of the extant Hippocratic works. Therefore, Galen has no reason to include Hippocrates as one of these 'ancient physicians' who name types of black bile differently like this. What we find in Galen's writing is that he adopts a pragmatic approach and in most cases he does not choose a consistent naming convention to differentiate systematically between various forms of black bile in his writing. Therefore, in a lot of cases we will find the term μέλαινα χολή, but sometimes it will be necessary for him to use the term μελαγχολικός χυμός or even 'melancholic blood' (μελαγχολικόν αἷμα). This will be the case when he has

---

8　　Just like in the case for 'acid', the reference here to the 'corrosive' (ξυστικός) nature of this
　　type of black bile is not what we think of as a corrosive chemical, but instead is related to
　　the way that this substance effervesces when in contact with the earth. See Siegel, 1968:
　　259–260.

9　　The translation of the passage from *On the Natural Faculties* by Brock above refers to differ-
　　ent portions or parts of the black bile humour. This allows Galen to differentiate between
　　two substances that have very different properties, but are closely related through the
　　action of heat on the 'according to nature' black bile to produce the 'contrary to nature'
　　black bile. We find in the passage above that Galen uses a unified view of black bile that
　　has different forms depending on the presence of extreme heat. This is useful for Galen, as
　　it allows him to combine the content relating to a single concept of black bile in the Hip-
　　pocratic *On the Nature of Man* with the different observations and descriptions of black
　　bile in other sources. However, as we have already seen in *On Affected Parts* and *On Black
　　Bile*, Galen sometimes does not emphasise the unified black bile because he is more con-
　　cerned with making clear distinctions between different types of black bile. We shall see
　　that the context of Galen's treatise, or even part of his treatise, is important to understand
　　the way that he is presenting black bile, either as a unified substance with different parts,
　　or as different substances that share a similar name. My use of the term 'type' here, rather
　　than 'portion' or 'part', allows me to differentiate between the 'according to nature' and
　　'contrary to nature' states of black bile and is compatible with my more general use of
　　terms for the different forms of black bile in this book.

10　　This passage is included by van der Eijk in the fragments that can be attributed to the
　　work of Diocles: See F27[12] (van der Eijk) = Gal. *Nat. Fac.* II.9 (II 134–136 K). See van der
　　Eijk, 2001: 49–53. I say that it is possible that Diocles made this distinction, as we can-
　　not completely rely on Galen's testimony of Diocles' terminology of black bile without an
　　independent reference to Diocles' actual writing on this subject.

to distinguish between the different kinds of black bile in a particular text for his specific argument. However, what is clear from the passage in *On the Natural Faculties* above is that different types of black bile can be distinguished by their ability to harm the body. We have seen that Galen has differentiated between them using the terms κατὰ φύσιν and παρὰ φύσιν. I now want to investigate further why this distinction is important for understanding Galen's characterisation of different forms of black bile.

These two terms κατὰ φύσιν and παρὰ φύσιν are very common and widespread in ancient medical literature and generally refer to the distinction between something that occurs naturally in the body as part of its normal function, in contrast to something that inhibits or has a negative effect on the health of the body, such as an external factor like too much heat or cold in the body. For example, we can find a definition of κατὰ φύσιν in *On the Doctrines of Hippocrates and Plato*:

> And as the term 'according to nature' is used in many ways, we must here take it to be used of that which occurs through the agency of nature in the first instance. By 'that which occurs through the agency of nature in the first instance' I mean that which nature seeks as an end, and not that which necessarily follows something else.[11]

In this passage, Galen tells us that κατὰ φύσιν can have many different meanings. Therefore, in order to put this term into context, he provides a specific example. So, we have a case where 'activity' (ἐνέργεια) is classified as being κατὰ φύσιν. This is then contrasted with the term for 'affection' (πάθος), which is said to be παρὰ φύσιν. In this way, Galen is using κατὰ φύσιν and παρὰ φύσιν to explain the difference between two related phenomena, where one is acting naturally, and the other unnaturally, based on its originally defined purpose.[12] We have seen earlier that Galen uses a teleological framework to explain that all parts of the body have been designed by 'Nature' for their purpose and function.[13] This

---

11 πολλαχῶς δὲ τοῦ κατὰ φύσιν λεγομένου, τοῦτ' ἀκούειν χρὴ νῦν ὃ κατὰ πρῶτον λόγον ὑπὸ τῆς φύσεως γίγνεται. κατὰ πρῶτον δὲ λόγον ἐκεῖνα γίγνεσθαί φαμεν ὑπὸ τῆς φύσεως, ὧν ὥσπερ σκοπῶν ἀντιποιεῖται καὶ μὴ δι' ἀκολουθίαν τινὰ ἑτέροις ἐξ ἀνάγκης ἕπεται. Galen, *PHP*, VI.1.8–9, CMG V 4,1,2, p. 362,5–8 De Lacy (V 507,9–16 K), translation by De Lacy. See Jouanna, 2002b: 234–235.

12 In *PHP* (VI.1.10–30, CMG V 4,1,2, p. 362,10–30 De Lacy (V 507,18–509,7 K)), Galen uses the example of the heart pulsating within itself as ἐνέργεια, but when the heart undergoes a palpitation, this is πάθος. See Jouanna, 2002b: 235–236.

13 See chapter 2, section 1 above.

applies to the presence and function of black bile in the body and also allows
Galen to make a distinction between conditions when black bile is functioning
κατὰ φύσιν and when it is acting παρὰ φύσιν.

I am going to consider two different ways that 'according to nature' (κατὰ
φύσιν) and 'contrary to nature' (παρὰ φύσιν) can be used in Galen's presentation
of the humours. Firstly, by applying these two terms to the humours, we can differentiate between different categories. For example in the case of phlegm, we
find the following:

> For it is not possible that this is not hot and dry, or hot and moist, or cold
> and dry, or cold and moist but inasmuch as it is to the greatest degree thick
> and cold, it falls outside the form of phlegm that accords with nature and
> rather seems to be another humour in the whole class contrary to nature.
> But this is definitely not the case. For if any [humour] is moist and cold
> in capacity, it is encompassed within the class of phlegm.[14]

In this passage from *On the Causes of Diseases*, we can see that there is a general
class of the humour 'phlegm', which is defined by the pairing of the cold and
moist qualities. However, there can be many different variations, such as being
thicker, colder, or wetter within this class. There is also an 'ideal' form of phlegm
that has the proper balance of the qualities that define it as being 'phlegm'.
There are other types of phlegm that may be thicker, colder or wetter than the
'ideal' phlegm, but as long as they possess the pairing of 'cold and moist' qualities, they are still classified as κατὰ φύσιν phlegm, although not the 'ideal' form.
However, if there is a loss of this pairing of 'cold and moist', then the substance
can no longer be considered κατὰ φύσιν, and is a παρὰ φύσιν type of phlegm.
This could occur if phlegm were heated or dried out. If we apply this model to
black bile, then any kind of black bile that has the pairing of qualities 'cold and
dry' comes under the category of κατὰ φύσιν black bile. The ideal form of black
bile is the innate humour that is described in the Hippocratic *On the Nature of
Man*. However, Galen's sediment, muddy and lees of blood forms of black bile
are also κατὰ φύσιν black bile, as these substances have the 'cold and dry' pairing
along with the other key properties of black bile, such as thickness. In contrast,
as we have seen in the passage from *On the Natural Faculties* quoted earlier (see

---

14 οὐ γὰρ ἐνδέχεται μὴ οὐχὶ θερμὸν εἶναι καὶ ξηρὸν αὐτὸν, ἢ θερμὸν καὶ ὑγρὸν, ἢ ψυχρὸν καὶ ξηρὸν, ἢ
    ψυχρὸν καὶ ὑγρόν, ἀλλ' ὅσον ἐπὶ πλεῖστον ἥκει πάχους καὶ ψύξεως, ἐκπίπτει μὲν τοῦ κατὰ φύσιν
    φλέγματος τῆς ἰδέας, ἕτερος δὲ εἶναι δοκεῖ χυμὸς ὅλῳ τῷ γένει παρὰ φύσιν. οὐ μὴν οὕτως γε ἔχει
    τἀληθές. ὅστις ἂν γὰρ ὑγρὸς ᾖ καὶ ψυχρὸς τὴν δύναμιν, ἐν τῷ τοῦ φλέγματος γένει περιέχεται.
    Caus. Morb. VI.3 (VII 22,14–23,3 K), translation by Johnston.

page 79 above), the acidic form of black bile that is produced by combustion or putrefaction has changed its form and faculty, resulting in the loss of its 'cold' quality, and therefore is classed as being παρὰ φύσιν black bile. So, Galen's use of κατὰ φύσιν and παρὰ φύσιν is one of the ways that he can distinguish between categories of black bile on the basis of their qualitative properties. This applies to the way that Galen describes black bile as one of the four humours that is present naturally in the body in *On the Elements According to Hippocrates*.[15]

Another way to interpret Galen's use of κατὰ φύσιν and παρὰ φύσιν is in the context of the humours 'acting' either 'according to nature' or 'contrary to nature'. This is related to the more general description of health and disease. For example in *On the Art of Medicine*, Galen defines good health as being κατὰ φύσιν and sickness as παρὰ φύσιν. This context of health and disease from the concept of κατὰ φύσιν and παρὰ φύσιν is also found in the Hippocratic Corpus, for example in *Prognostic* and *On the Nature of Man*.[16] This idea of a natural state can also be used to define any deviation of a humour that can lead to illness and disease. This movement away from what is natural brings in the term παρὰ φύσιν, which describes an unnatural state of a humour. We can see this in Galen's *On the Causes of Symptoms* where there is a more general description of the way that the humours can 'act' contrary to nature and so cause harm in the body:

> Colours, then, will be changed, to speak briefly, as a result of humours departing from their natural form, or sinking down to the depths, or over-flowing, as it were, the skin, but in specific cases as a result of causes compelling the humours to come to such movements and conditions. There are, of course, the psychical affections and the changes of the air surrounding us towards hot or cold. And there are conditions of the body itself, which has its blood hotter, or colder, or less or more, or pushed to the exterior, or drawn to the interior. Of this class also is every bad humour which changes the colour of the whole body according to its own form, in jaundice, dropsy, elephas and weaknesses of the spleen and liver. Analogous too are the discolorations which will arise in relation to any part

---

15 For example: *Hipp. Elem.* 8.14; 13.3, CMG V 1,2, pp. 126,15–16; 148,20–22 De Lacy (I 480,11–13; 502,1–4 K). See also *PHP*, VIII.5.27; 35, CMG V 4,1,2, pp. 510,10; 512,4–5 De Lacy (V 685,10–11; 687,9–10 K).

16 Gal. *Ars. Med.* XXI (I 358,7–9 K); Hippocratic Corpus, *Prog.* X (II 134,5 L); *Nat. Hom.* 2, CMG I 1,3, p. 168,5–8 Jouanna (VI 36,1–4 L). Jouanna points out that Galen also introduces an intermediary state (ἐν μεθορίῳ) between κατὰ φύσιν and παρα φύσιν, which is not found in the extant Hippocratic Corpus. See Jouanna, 2002b: 241.

whatever. And the natural forms will be changed when the parts are filled
or evacuated more excessively, or removed from their particular place, or
forcibly drawn aside.[17]

This passage tells us that Galen postulated that it is possible for the humours to
'change' from their κατά φύσιν state and cause disease in the body. This is supported by a similar statement in *On the Art of Medicine*, where we find that the
humours can 'deviate' into states that are παρά φύσιν and harm the body, such as
causing disease in the liver and other organs.[18] If we investigate the Hippocratic
Corpus, we can see a similar idea of κατά φύσιν used to define the four humours,
as being substances that always remain the same in accordance with nature.[19]
When it comes to the opposing term, παρά φύσιν, there is only one instance of it
in *On the Nature of Man*, and this defines the ability of the four humours to produce disease through the effects of their innate qualities, by heating, cooling,
drying and moistening.[20] This definition of κατά φύσιν and παρά φύσιν can help
us understand how the innate black bile humour can cause disease in the body.
The innate form of black bile is natural, essential and is produced from the very
beginning of life and performs a necessary part of the overall humoral mixture
to maintain health in the body. However, it can act παρά φύσιν if it causes disease in the body by either being in excess in relation to the proper humoral
mixture, or becomes separated from the mixture to settle in some part of the
body. The same situation applies to the sediment, muddy and lees of blood
types of black bile, which we have seen can be also classified as κατά φύσιν,

---

17   χρώματα μὲν οὖν ὑπαλλαχθήσεται, συνελόντι μὲν εἰπεῖν, διὰ τοὺς χυμοὺς ἐξισταμένους τῆς κατὰ
      φύσιν ἰδέας, ἢ ὑπονοστοῦντας εἰς τὸ βάθος, ἢ οἷον ἐπικλύζοντας τὸ δέρμα κατὰ μέρος δὲ, διὰ τὰς
      τοὺς χυμοὺς ἀναγκαζούσας αἰτίας εἰς τὰς τοιαύτας ἀφικνεῖσθαι κινήσεις τε καὶ διαθέσεις. ἔστι
      δὲ δήπου τὰ πάθη τὰ ψυχικὰ καὶ τοῦ περιέχοντος ἡμᾶς ἀέρος αἱ εἰς θερμότητά τε καὶ ψυχρό-
      τητα μεταβολαί. καὶ αὐτοῦ τοῦ σώματος γὰρ αἱ διαθέσεις, ἢ θερμότερον ἴσχοντος, ἢ ψυχρότερον,
      ἢ ἔλαττον, ἢ πλέον, ἢ ὠθούμενον ἐκτός, ἢ ἀντισπώμενον ἔσω τὸ αἷμα. τούτου δ' ἐστὶ τοῦ γένους
      καὶ ἡ κακοχυμία πᾶσα, κατὰ τὴν ἑαυτῆς ἰδέαν ἀλλοιοῦσα καὶ τὴν ἅπαντος τοῦ σώματος χροιάν,
      ἐν ἰκτέροις τε καὶ ὑδέροις καὶ ἐλέφασι καὶ σπληνὸς καὶ ἥπατος ἀτονίαις. ἀνάλογον δὲ καὶ αἱ καθ'
      ὁτιοῦν μόριον ἄχροιαι συστήσονται. τὰ δὲ κατὰ φύσιν ὑπαλλαχθήσεται σχήματα, πληρουμένων
      ἀμετρότερον, ἢ κενουμένων τῶν μορίων, ἢ τῆς οἰκείας χώρας μεθισταμένων, ἢ παρασπωμένων.
      Symp. Caus. XII.1 (VII 267,9–268 K), translation by Johnston.
18   For example, *Ars. Med.* 19 (I 356,4–5 K).
19   *Nat. Hom.* 5, CMG I 1,3, pp. 174,11–176,1 Jouanna (VI 40,15–17 L). At the same point in the
      text the author also defines the four humours as remaining the same in accordance with
      convention (κατὰ νόμον).
20   *Nat. Hom.* 2, CMG I 1,3, p. 168,6–8 (VI 36,1–4 L). However, I cannot find any examples in the
      extant Hippocratic Corpus where παρά φύσιν is applied directly to the definition of black
      bile.

but are considered to be the cause of diseases such as melancholy and quartan fevers.[21] But, these types of black bile are only acting παρὰ φύσιν, they are not themselves 'contrary to nature' substances. However, the acidic type of black bile is a παρὰ φύσιν state and so is itself 'contrary to nature' and is not part of the class of the natural black bile humour that is 'cold and dry'. Instead, this is a case where substances, such as black bile or yellow bile, have undergone a transformation of their actual form and faculty to become a black substance with acidic and corrosive properties, which is extremely harmful to the body. This substance will cause damage to the bodily tissue and will produce disease in the body. Therefore, if a physician identifies that it is present in the body, it must be removed as quickly as possible, or the patient may die. This classification of black bile, as κατὰ φύσιν and παρὰ φύσιν, is also useful when it comes to explaining what appears to be a potential inconsistency in Galen's qualitative characterisation of the black bile humour.

2 A Question of Consistency in Galen's Qualitative Characterisation of Black Bile

We have seen that Galen has postulated different forms of the black bile humour in order to explain how various types of disease can occur and he does this by drawing upon a wider set of sources than the one type of black bile characterised in *On the Nature of Man*. However, Galen's use of various terms and descriptions for black bile in different treatises might be viewed as a possible source of inconsistency in his writing. This very question of consistency has been raised by Jouanna, who compares passages from *On the Natural Faculties* and *On Black Bile*. The material from *On the Natural Faculties* describes black bile as a 'cold and dry' humour, which is predominant in autumn, and is generally linked to a particular time of life, regimes and climates that are cold and dry. This is consistent with the characterisation of black bile that we find in the Hippocratic *On the Nature of Man*.[22] However, Jouanna has identified the following passage from *On Black Bile* as a potential problem for Galen's writing on black bile:

> Hippocrates says that its [black bile] production is necessary, but he advised on how it might not be produced in excess, beginning his advice

---

21   See chapter 7, sections 1 and 2 below.

22   *Nat. Fac.* II.9 (II 130,15–131,9 K). See Siegel, 1968: 238; Jouanna, 2009: 238–239.

with examples that were clearly visible. More black bile seems to be produced in living beings which are hotter and drier in temperament, and
also at hotter and drier times of the year, and in hotter and drier places
and constitutions, and in patterns of life that are wrapped in depression,
stress and insomnia, and of the driest foods that consist of thick particles.[23]

The question that Jouanna poses is: if black bile is a 'cold and dry' humour,
how is it possible for it to flourish in conditions that are 'hot and dry'? Jouanna
reports that there has been some concern about the presence of this description of black bile, which is defined as being produced in 'hot and dry' conditions. It is Jouanna's opinion that this has caused there to be a 'tendency for
this characterisation to be unconsciously erased' (*que l'on a tendance à gommer
inconsciemment*) from our thoughts about the nature of black bile in Galen's
writing.[24] However, my analysis of the way that Galen purposely characterises
different types of black bile offers an alternative view to understand more about
how Galen distinguishes between different types of black bile that have very
different physical properties.

We saw from the passage in *On the Natural Faculties*, which I quoted earlier
(see page 79 above), that the 'contrary to nature' (παρὰ φύσιν) black bile can be
produced from the 'combustion' (σύγκαυσις) of the 'according to nature' (κατὰ
φύσιν) black bile. However, if we investigate Galen's writing on black bile more
generally, we find that in the presence of a 'hot and dry' condition in the body,
black bile can be produced from the burning of different substances, not just
the κατὰ φύσιν black bile, but other humours as well.[25] From now on, I am going
to refer to κατὰ φύσιν black bile as 'natural black bile' and παρὰ φύσιν black bile
as 'altered black bile'. This part of Galen's theory of black bile is complicated
because we find slightly different explanations for the production of black bile
in a range of treatises. So far, from *On the Natural Faculties*, we know that a
transformation occurs due to the heating of natural black bile to create the
altered black bile with its acidic properties. If we move on to *On Black Bile*, we
find the following statement by Galen:

---

23   ἣν Ἱπποκράτης φησὶν ἀναγκαίαν μὲν ἔχειν τὴν γένεσιν, ὅπως δὲ μὴ γένοιτο πλείων, ἐδίδαξεν ἐξ
      αὐτῶν τῶν ἐναργῶς φαινομένων ἀρξάμενος. ἔν τε γὰρ τοῖς ζῴοις, ὅσα θερμότερα καὶ ξηρότερα
      ταῖς κράσεσιν, φαίνεται γεννᾶσθαι πλέον, ἔν τε ταῖς θερμοτέραις ἅμα καὶ ξηροτέραις ὥραις τε καὶ
      χώραις καὶ καταστάσεσιν, ἐπιτηδεύμασί τε τοῖς μετὰ κόπων καὶ φροντίδων καὶ ἀγρυπνιῶν, ἐδε-
      σμάτων τε τῶν παχυμερῶν καὶ ξηροτάτων. *At. Bil.* 6, CMG V 4,1,1, p. 82,9–16 De Boer (V 126,1–11
      κ), adapted from a translation by Grant.
24   Jouanna, 2009: 242–243 and 250.
25   Siegel, 1968: 219.

Its [black bile's] formation therefore appears to be destructive, the result of the black humour being heated too much. You must remember, of course, that black bile which results from an excessive heating of yellow bile is more destructive than the black bile I mentioned before, just as one humour is more drastic in its action compared with another humour; such as yellow bile [compared with] sediment of blood.[26]

In this passage Galen refers to two different forms of altered black bile. One type is formed from the heating of the black humour (μέλας χυμός), which, as we have seen from the passage in *On the Natural Faculties* above (page 79), is the black bile that resembles sediment or lees in blood. The other kind of altered black bile comes from the heating of yellow bile. However, if we investigate other texts by Galen, we find a slight change in the way that he describes which substances are heated to produce black bile. For example in *Commentary on Prorrhetics I*, *Commentary on Epidemics* and *Commentary on Aphorisms*, there are clear statements about a dual production of black bile, either from the roasting of yellow bile or thick blood.[27] There are two ways to interpret what Galen means by thick blood here. One is that he is referring to a thicker type of the pure blood humour. This is plausible, as Galen does discuss the presence of a thicker and thinner type of the pure blood humour in *On Black Bile*. The other possibility is that Galen actually means the thick part of the composite blood, which is due to the presence of the natural black bile in the humoral mixture.[28]

However, what we find is that both types of substance, pure blood and natural black bile in blood, are used by Galen when he refers to the production of altered black bile by combustion. I will start with the evidence that it is the natural black bile in blood, which is heated to produce altered black bile. We

---

26   καὶ διὰ τοῦτο ἔοικεν ἡ γένεσις αὐτῆς ὀλέθριος ὑπάρχειν ὑπεροπτηθέντος τοῦ μέλανος χυμοῦ συμβαίνουσα. πολὺ δὲ δήπου τῆς δε τὴν ἐκ τῆς ξανθῆς χολῆς ὑπεροπτηθείσης γινομένην μέλαιναν ὀλεθριωτέραν εἶναι νομιστέον, ὥσπερ καὶ ὁ χυμὸς τοῦ χυμοῦ δραστικώτερος, ἡ ξανθὴ χολὴ τῆς οἷον ὑποστάθμης τοῦ αἵματος. *At. Bil.* 3, CMG V 4,1,1, p. 75,6–12 De Boer (V 112,1–6 K), adapted from a translation by Grant.

27   *Hipp. Prorrh.* I.4, CMG V 9,2, p. 14,18–22 Diels (XVI 512,11–16 K); *Hipp. Epid.* VI.VI.3, CMG V 10,2,2, p. 328,8–10 Wenkebach (XVIIb 321,18–322,2 K); *Hipp. Aph.* III.22 (XVIIb 622,4–6 K). See Joanna, 2009: 249.

28   *At. Bil.*, 2, CMG V 4,1,1, p. 72,23 De Boer (V 107,4–5 K). Jouanna takes the first case, which implies that Galen has developed a theory based on the production of black bile from the excessive heating of yellow bile or blood in these treatises. He suggests that in *On the Natural Faculties*, Galen had only mentioned the production of black bile from the combustion of either natural black bile or from yellow bile. Whereas, in *On Black Bile*, Galen's view is that black bile is produced from the roasting of yellow bile or blood. See Jouanna, 2009: 249–250.

have already seen in the passage from *On Black Bile*, quoted above, that Galen describes one of the substances that is heated as the 'sediment' (ὑποστάθμης) of blood. We know that this is the type of characterisation of black bile that Galen uses for his description of black bile. Further to this, in *Commentary on Prognostic*, Galen refers to the thick part of the blood as like the 'lees of wine' (τῶν οἴνων τρυγὶ); again we have seen that this is how Galen characterises black bile.[29] On the other hand, there are examples where Galen seems to be discussing the heating of the pure blood humour. For example, in *On Mixtures*, we find the following: '... just as one who was previously hot and dry has produced a very great quantity of black bile from the burning of his blood'.[30] In this treatise, Galen describes 'melancholic mixtures' (μελαγχολικαὶ κράσεις), which are produced from the extreme heat of the blood in the body. This is part of Galen's criticism of anyone who thinks that all very hairy people are melancholic. He explains that the mixture of the hot and dry qualities in the body that causes the growth of hair is not the same process that creates a melancholic condition in the body. Instead, the melancholic mixtures are produced by an incomplete combustion of the blood.[31] There is also a passage in Galen's *On the Causes of Symptoms*, where he discusses the way that black bile might be produced from blood:

> For blood that has been cooled does not generate black bile, as in the case of a clot, but when overheated has, on this account also, a preserved brightness. For black bile also has a genesis in this way, not like a clot, which is blood that has been cooled. On the contrary, black bile like ash arises entirely from overheating and boiling. It is cold in that it is earth-like, but partakes of heat as do ash and vinegar.[32]

The part about the clotting of blood is reminiscent of Galen's explanation in *On Black Bile* of the way to identify black blood, which has an ability to congeal

---

29   *Hipp. Prog.* III.32, CMG V 9,2, p. 356,4–11 Heeg (XVIIIb 278,4–13 K). See Jouanna, 2009: 249 (note 35).

30   ... οἷον εἴ τις ἔμπροσθεν ὑπάρχων θερμὸς καὶ ξηρὸς ἐκ συγκαύσεως τοῦ αἵματος πλείστην ἐγέν-νησε τὴν μέλαιναν χολήν. *Temp.* II.6 (I 643,1–3 K), translation by Singer.

31   *Temp.* II.6 (I 641,4–643,9 K).

32   οὐ γὰρ ἀποψυχόμενον τὸ αἷμα γεννᾷ τὴν μέλαιναν χολήν, ὥσπερ ἐπὶ τοῦ θρόμβου, ἀλλ᾽ ὑπερο-πτώμενον, διὸ καὶ τὴν στιλπνότητα διασωζομένην ἔχει. οὐ γὰρ ὡς ὁ θρόμβος, ἀποψυχθέντος τοῦ αἵματος, οὕτω καὶ ἡ μέλαινα χολὴ τὴν γένεσιν ἔχει· τοὐναντίον γὰρ ἅπαν ἐξ ὑπεροπτήσεώς τε καὶ ζέσεως, οἷον τέφρα τις ἡ μέλαινα χολὴ συνίσταται, ψυχρὰ μὲν, ὅτι γεώδης, θερμότητος δὲ μετέ-χουσα, καθάπερ ἡ τέφρα τε καὶ τὸ ὄξος. *Sympt. Caus.* VII.3 (VII 245,17–246,6 K), translation by Johnston. See Jouanna, 2009: 249 (note 35).

that black bile does not (see page 94 below).[33] This passage tells us that blood can be heated to the point that black bile is produced. In addition, the comparison with ash is like Galen's description of the burnt black bile at the end of the passage from *On the Natural Faculties* (see page 79 above), but this time the ashes retain both the qualities of 'cold' and 'hot'. The reference to vinegar provides the altered black bile with the property of acidity that we have seen already in *On the Natural Faculties* and *On Black Bile*.[34]

---

33   *At. Bil.* 3, CMG V 4,1,1, p. 74,16–17 De Boer (V 110,14–66 K).

34   For Jouanna, all these examples are part of what he considers to be an overall problem of inconsistency in the qualitative properties of black bile. This corresponds to the difference between the 'cold and dry' black bile in the Hippocratic *On the Nature of Man*, and the passages from Galen's treatises where black bile is produced in 'hot and dry' conditions. Jouanna's suggestion for a resolution to this apparent inconsistency can be found in Galen's *Commentary on On the Nature of Man*. Jouanna refers specifically to a passage from this text, where Galen makes the following remark: "And this [black bile] arises likewise from the humours being cooked during the summer. And what remains from the cooking, when the heat is clearly extinguished, then becomes cold and dry; cold on account of the heat being extinguished, dry because of all the wetness being driven off during the cooking." ἐγένετο δ' εἰκότως τοιοῦτος διὰ τὸ προκατωπτῆσθαι τοὺς χυμοὺς τῷ θέρει. τὸ δ' ὑπόλειμμα τῶν ὀπτηθέντων, ὅταν δηλονότι σβεσθῇ τὸ θερμόν, αὐτίκα γίνεται ψυχρόν τε καὶ ξηρόν, ψυχρὸν μὲν διὰ τὴν τοῦ θερμοῦ σβέσιν, ξηρὸν δέ, ὅτι κατὰ τὴν ὄπτησιν ἐξεδαπανήθη πᾶν τὸ ὑγρὸν ἐξ αὐτοῦ. (*HNH*, I.34, CMG V 9,1, p. 45,26–28 Mewaldt (XV 86,9–12 K), translation by Lewis.) According to Jouanna, this passage shows an attempt by Galen to resolve the issue of the difference between black bile in terms of the paired qualities 'cold and dry' and 'hot and dry'. This is because Galen shows that in summer ('hot and dry' environment) the humours become roasted and produce a residue that is the black bile humour. However, when the heat is gone, the residue becomes colder and so the resulting residue is cooled and becomes 'cold and dry'. He suggests that this is the place where Galen resolves the missing 'cold' quality that is absent in *On Black Bile*. Jouanna also brings in reference to the passages from *On the Causes of Symptoms*, which I quoted earlier, see page 88 above. Further to this, he refers to passages from *Hipp. Prog.* (II.46, CMG V 9.2, p. 297,4–5 (XVIIIb 175,16–176,2 K)) and *PHP* (VIII.4.21, CMG V 4,2,1, p. 502,22 De Lacy (V 676,15 K)) as similar examples where the traditional cold and earthy qualities are applied to black bile in this context. See Jouanna, 2009: 253–254. His conclusion is that Galen has developed an overall theory of black bile, which incorporates the innate, essential humoral black bile from the Hippocratic *On the Nature of Man*, with a 'blackened' and 'non-innate' form of black bile, which comes from the influence of another Hippocratic treatise, *Airs, Waters and Places*. See Jouanna, 2009: 254. The passage that Jouanna identifies is from the tenth section of this text: "For if the weather be northerly and dry, with no rain either during the Dog Star or at Arcturus, it is very beneficial to those who have a phlegmatic or humid constitution, and to women, but it is very harmful to the bilious. For these dry up overmuch, and are attacked by dry ophthalmia and by acute, protracted fevers, in some cases too by melancholies. For the most humid and watery part of the bile is dried up and is spent, while the thickest and most acrid part is left, and similarly with blood." Ἢν δὲ βόρειόν τε ᾖ καὶ ἄνυδρον, καὶ μήτε ὑπὸ κύνα ἔπομβρον, μήτε ἐπὶ τῷ ἀρκτούρῳ, τοῖσι μὲν φλεγματίῃσι φύσει ξυμφέρει

Jouanna attempts to resolve the apparent inconsistency between black bile as a 'cold and dry' substance in *On the Natural Faculties* and the production of black bile from a 'hot and dry' environment in *On Black Bile*. He argues that the distinction between the ideal form of humoral black bile and other types of black bile is not clearly defined in Galen's *On Black Bile* and so this is a mistake on Galen's part that he then had to put right. The result is that Galen attempted to address this inconsistency in his *Commentary on On the Nature of Man*, which Jouanna regards as being consistent with the content on black bile in the Hippocratic *On the Nature of Man*. But then Galen emphasises the restoration of the 'cold' quality to black bile by a cooling process, which occurs after the initial heating process that produced the harmful type of black bile. This provides the pathological black bile with the quality of 'cold', which Jouanna believes Galen had to reinstate because it is missing from his description in *On Black Bile*.[35]

μάλιστα, καὶ τοῖσιν ὑγροῖσι τὰς φύσιας, καὶ τῇσι γυναιξίν· τοῖσι δὲ χολώδεσι τοῦτο πολεμιώτατον γίγνεται· λίην γὰρ ἀναξηραίνονται, καὶ ὀφθαλμίαι αὐτέοισιν ἐπιγίγνονται ξηραὶ, καὶ πυρετοὶ ὀξέες καὶ πολυχρόνιοι, ἐνίοισι δὲ καὶ μελαγχολίαι. Τῆς γὰρ χολῆς τὸ μὲν ὑγρότατον καὶ ὑδαρέστατον ἀναλοῦται, τὸ δὲ παχύτατον καὶ δριμύτατον λείπεται, καὶ τοῦ αἵματος κατὰ τὸν αὐτὸν λόγον. *Aer.* X (II 50,6–14 L), translation by Jones. See Jouanna, 2009: 254 (note 44). We can see the reason for Jouanna's reference to this passage from *Airs, Waters and Places*, as the hot weather causes a heating and drying of bile and blood. However, there is no reference to the type of extreme heating or 'roasting' that Galen uses in his explanation that we have seen above. In addition, *Airs, Waters and Places*, although considered to be authentic by Galen, does not contain any explicit reference to the black bile humour itself. In fact, we only have this single instance of the term 'melancholies', which in Galen's medical theory is related to the presence of the black bile humour in the body. Further to this, Jouanna has identified another possible influence on Galen's development of black bile that is produced from the combustion of other substances. This time we go beyond the Hippocratic Corpus, to the work of Rufus of Ephesus. As Jouanna points out, Galen does refer to Rufus as one of the prominent physicians writing about black bile at the start of *On Black Bile*. Jouanna associates this material from the work of Rufus on melancholy with what Galen says in his *Commentary on On the Nature of Man* because of the similarity of the language used for the roasting and cooling of yellow bile. *At. Bil.* 1, CMG V 4,1,1, p. 71,12–14 De Boer (V 105,3–4 K). See Jouanna, 2009: 254–255. Jouanna refers to a passage attributed to Rufus, which reports that there are two types of melancholy, the second of which is caused by the excessive roasting of yellow bile, which is then described as being cooled after the extreme heating. Rufus of Ephesus, F11[22–24] (Pormann) = Aëtius, *Medical Books*, vi. 9 (frg. 70 (Daremberg)). See Jouanna, 2009: 255 (note 45). Aëtius of Amida (fl. c. 500–550 CE) composed the *Medical Books*, which contains a large amount of 'quotes' from Rufus' *On Melancholy*. See Pormann, 2008: 13.

35　Jouanna, 2009: 255–256. I agree that Galen had developed a theoretical model of black bile that incorporates the existence of a number of distinct versions of this humour. This is because Galen needed to distinguish between different types of black bile in order to account for cases where black bile functions as a humour that promotes health and also

However, I think there is an alternative view that Galen's strategy is to provide different arguments in the context of the treatises that we have discussed so far. Therefore, in both *On the Natural Faculties* and *On Black Bile*, Galen is creating a polemical argument against what he considers as the incorrect views of rivals, such as Erasistratus and his followers, on the subject of black bile. The difference between these two treatises is that Galen emphasises the description of black bile as a 'cold and dry' humour in *On the Natural Faculties* because it is useful to his argument against Erasistratus. In contrast, Galen does not need to mention that black bile has the quality of 'cold' in *On Black Bile* because it is not necessary for his argument in this treatise, which instead mostly concerns the harmful effect of altered black bile. In the case of Galen's commentaries on texts from the Hippocratic Corpus, we find that he is offering explanations and interpretations of what he considers to be Hippocrates' opinion on black bile. Therefore, when he is discussing *On the Nature of Man* in his commentary, he is engaging with what is actually in this text. This means that he writes about the combustion of the other humours to produce black bile, as if this is what Hippocrates meant when he wrote the section on the predominance of the humours in different seasons. In the other commentaries, Galen takes the opportunity to explain the texts based on his view of the production of the altered form of black bile from the combustion of natural black bile, yellow bile or blood. Again, Galen's strategy is to interpret the text, as if this is what Hippocrates originally meant to say. The pairing of qualities are retained by Galen throughout, as the natural black bile is 'cold and dry' and the altered black bile is changed in its form and faculty to become acidic and hot. Here the altered black bile gains the capacity of 'hotness', which is why it can no longer be classified as natural black bile. However, Galen explains that in some circumstances the natural form of black bile, which is 'cold and dry', can be created, or that

---

when black bile is harmful to the body and causes disease. We can see that one particular form of black bile is produced when the humours, natural black bile, yellow bile or blood become extremely heated in the body. I agree also with the idea that Galen is attempting to bring together material relating to both of these types of black bile from a wide variety of sources, such as *On the Nature of Man*, *Airs, Waters and Places*, and other material such as the cause of melancholy attributed to Rufus of Ephesus. However, I disagree with Jouanna's conclusion relating to the superiority of the characterisation of black bile in the *Commentary on On the Nature of Man* and *On the Natural Faculties* in comparison with that of *On Black Bile*. In my opinion, this puts too much emphasis on the Hippocratic *On the Nature of Man*, as the most important basis for Galen's development of his theory of the black bile humour. I do not think that it is necessary to try to resolve this apparent inconsistency between the characterisation of black bile as 'cold and dry' and 'hot and dry' in Galen's writing.

the 'cold and dry' qualities are restored to the altered form of black bile. The latter can occur in the situations where the extreme heat is removed, and there is a cooling process. However, on this final point Galen is not so consistent or precise, which is the result of his flexibility of using slightly different characterisations of black bile in various arguments. However, I think that Galen was well aware of what he was doing, as I do not believe that he was concerned too much about this issue of apparent inconsistency between different types of black bile in regards to the qualities. Instead, I believe that Galen's main focus for writing about black bile in this way is within the context of providing physicians with the information necessary to identify and treat medical conditions that involve the presence of large amounts of black bile in the body. For Galen, this was particularly important when the altered form of black bile is present in the body.

3   Summary

We have seen that Galen has differentiated between three main types of black bile, but in order to understand how he uses them in his writing on health and disease in the body, it is important to investigate the way that he differentiates between them by name. We have found that Galen can be more or less strict about the proper naming of these three types of black bile. He is clear in *On Affected Parts*, when he names the innate form 'black bile' (μέλαινα χολή) and the sediment, lees-like or mud-like black bile 'melancholic humour' (μελαγχολικὸς χυμός) or 'melancholic blood' (μελαγχολικόν αἷμα). However, he also refers to the acidic form of black bile as μελαγχολικὸς χυμός. Galen claims that, although some people incorrectly use the term μελαγχολικὸς χυμός for both, he can use the same name as he understands the important distinctions between these two types of black bile. But there is an added complexity, as Galen also refers to the sediment, mud-like, lees-like and acidic forms as μέλαινα χολή in treatises such as *On Mixtures* and *On the Therapeutic Method*. This is because in the earlier medical and philosophical sources that Galen draws upon, such as the Hippocratic Corpus and the writing of Plato and the Aristotelians, the term μέλαινα χολή is far more common than μελαγχολικὸς χυμός. Galen's application of what he calls 'loose language' is his preferred stance, as it is more flexible for him to incorporate and discuss many different sources for his writing on black bile. Therefore, it is more useful for Galen's strategy to incorporate a wide range of sources and show that there is agreement between them. We also found that Galen classified the different types of black bile on the basis of the two terms 'according to nature' (κατὰ φύσιν) and 'contrary to nature' (παρὰ φύσιν).

Both the innate black bile and the sediment, mud-like or lees-like black bile come under the category of κατὰ φύσιν, as they all are defined by the pairing of 'cold and dry' qualities. However, the difference between them is that the innate black bile represents the ideal natural form, as it has the perfect blend of cold and dry, along with other important qualities such as its thickness and colour. The sediment, mud-like and lees-like forms are non-ideal states of natural black bile, as their qualities deviate from the perfect balance of the ideal black bile. Therefore, in order to distinguish between them, I will refer to the innate form as 'ideal natural black bile' and the sediment, mud-like and lees-like forms collectively as 'non-ideal natural black bile'. The acidic forms of black bile are classified as παρὰ φύσιν because their qualities are altered from what is found in the natural state of black bile. Therefore, I will refer to the different types of black bile that are produced from the extreme heating of the humours collectively as 'altered black bile'. This analysis is useful because it can help to explain why there appears to be inconsistencies in Galen's writing on black bile. For example, the possible issue of the difference in the characterisation of black bile between *On the Natural Faculties* and *On Black Bile* can be resolved by considering the context of Galen's argument in each of these treatises. This provides an alternative explanation for the absence of the 'cold' quality in Galen's description of black bile in *On Black Bile* because he is referring to the harmful type of black bile that is 'hot'. The way that Galen writes about the various forms of black bile in different treatises is essential for our understanding of how this humour is used to provide information on health and disease in the body. We shall see in the next chapter that Galen emphasises the importance of the altered black bile because it is so harmful to the body.

CHAPTER 5

Galen's Explanation of Harmful Black Bile

In the last chapter we found that Galen differentiated between three different forms of black bile, two which are classified as being 'according to nature' and a type of black bile that acts 'contrary to nature' in the body. I have named this latter form 'altered black bile' and in order to understand Galen's writing on this humour, it is important to know more about the way that he characterises this very harmful type of black bile in different treatises.

1 The Properties of Altered Black Bile and How This Makes It a Potentially Harmful Substance in the Body

The altered type of black bile is very important in Galen's biological theory of the cause of disease because it has specific harmful properties, which we have already seen in a passage from *On the Natural Faculties* quoted above (page 79). Here we found that Galen described altered black bile on the basis of its acridity (ξυστικὸν) and corrosive effects (ὀξώδη), along with fermentation and bubbling (ζύμωσίν τε καὶ ζέσιν). This is in contrast to natural black bile, which does not produce the seething and fermentation on the ground (ζέσιν τε καὶ ζύμωσιν τῆς γῆς). The reason why this information is so essential for Galen is that it can be used to tell the difference between substances found in evacuated material, such as vomit and faeces. For example, Galen provides guidance on how to distinguish between black bile and other black compounds in *On Black Bile*:

> Therefore, because [black bile] cannot be congealed, it can be distinguished from the black blood, but not from anything particularly named black. For such a thing often is vomited and is excreted through the bowels and is very much different from black bile, not only in its capacity, but in its perceptible qualities. For clearly such a thing shares neither of the sourness nor acridity of black bile, which exhibits [these properties], by way of the taste for those who vomit and by way of smell, not only for that person, but for all those [around him]. Nor does it cause effervescence with the ground, as black bile does.[1]

---

1 Ὅτι μὲν οὖν οὐ πήγνυται, διώρισται μὲν ἀπὸ τοῦ μέλανος αἵματος, οὐ μὴν ἤδη γε καὶ ἀπὸ τῶν μελά-

© KONINKLIJKE BRILL NV, LEIDEN, 2019 | DOI:10.1163/9789004382794_007

The issue raised by Galen here is about the ability to distinguish between substances coming out of the body that all appear to be black. The first comparison that Galen makes is between black blood and altered black bile. Now black blood will be liquid at first and then will congeal in the way that it can be seen to do naturally. However, Galen remarks that altered black bile can be distinguished from this blood, as it does not congeal in this way. This is supported by a similar argument that Galen makes when he provides information on the way to distinguish black blood from altered black bile in his *Commentary on Aphorisms*. Just as in the previous example, black blood is distinct, as it pours forth (κεχύσθαι) and is congealed (πεπηγέναι). In contrast, altered black bile when poured, solidifies apart (χωρὶς πεπῆχθαι), which is different from the way that blood congeals. The resultant altered black bile has a shiny black appearance (τῷ στίλβον ἔχειν τὸ μέλαν), is pungent like vinegar (δακνῶδες εἶναι καθάπερ ὄξος) and importantly reacts with the earth to form bubbles (ζυμοῦν τὴν γῆν).[2] We have seen that *Aphorisms* was considered by Galen to be one of the best examples (alongside *Prognostic* and *Epidemics I* and *III*) of Hippocrates' writing. We find that Galen is describing altered black bile when he is interpreting these passages from *Aphorisms*. This is important because Galen is able to draw the reader towards the conclusion that Hippocrates is in agreement with the existence of this altered black bile, which Galen wants to use in his biological theory. However, there are no other comparisons between black blood and black bile relating to being congealed (πήγνυται) in any of the other extant Galenic treatises, or in the extant Hippocratic Corpus. So it appears from what we have on his work that Galen has only raised this issue of the difference of coagulation between black bile and black blood in *On Black Bile* and in his commentary on a passage from the Hippocratic *Aphorisms*.

The inability to congeal also applies to the other black non-blood substances in vomit and faeces. So, as we see in the passage quoted above from *On Black*

νων ἰδίως ὀνομαζομένων. ἐμεῖταί τε γὰρ καὶ διαχωρεῖται πολλάκις τοιαῦτα πάμπολυ διαφέροντα τῆς μελαίνης χολῆς οὐ τῇ δυνάμει μόνον, ἀλλὰ καὶ ταῖς αἰσθηταῖς ποιότησιν. οὔτε γὰρ στρυφνότητος οὔτε ὀξύτητος μετέχει σαφῶς ταῦτα τῆς μελαίνης χολῆς κατά τε τὴν γεῦσιν ἐμφαινούσης τοῖς ἐμοῦσιν αὐτὴν καὶ κατὰ τὴν ὄσφρησιν οὐκ ἐκείνοις μόνον, ἀλλὰ καὶ τοῖς ἄλλοις. οὐ μὴν οὐδὲ ζυμοῖ τὴν γῆν, ὡς ἐκείνη. *At. Bil.* 3, CMG V 4,1,1, p. 74,16–23 De Boer (V 110,14–111,6 K), adapted from a translation by Grant.

2 *Hipp. Aph.* IV.23 (XVIIb 687,1–688,4 K). At this point Galen is referring to the parts of the Hippocratic *Aphorisms* (IV.21–23 (IV 508,5–510,7 L)) that have observations of evacuated matter during different types of illness. These substances can be described as being black; sometimes they seem like black blood, black bile, or simply black matter. Galen stresses the importance for the physician to be able to accurately tell the difference, as this affects diagnosis and prognosis of the illness.

Bile, the way to tell whether the black substances are black bile or not can be determined from their effect on the body and from their odour. So Galen says that the black matter can be distinguished from what is actually altered black bile, because it does not have the same 'bite' (δῆξις) or produce the unpleasant smell (ὀσμὴν δυσώδη) that is associated with altered black bile.[3] In addition, altered black bile has a distinct sourness (στρυφνότητος) and acridity (ὀξύτητος), which can be detected by taste and smell. Galen is particularly concerned about the possibility of a similarity between vinegar and altered black bile, which could lead to a misidentification of altered black bile and so he provides advice on how to tell the difference between them in *On Black Bile*:

> But if according to this, black bile appears similar to very acidic vinegar, it is constituted with thick particles completely opposite of the substance [of vinegar], when it is neat in contact with parts of the body, it ulcerates and corrodes the body in all ways. For the vinegar, seeing that it is composed of fine particles, it passes through [the body], but the thickness of the black bile provides lasting resting places for it which becomes the cause of the corrosion.[4]

So, altered black bile may be similar to very sharp vinegar based on acidity, but very different in its structure. For his description of altered black bile, Galen uses the term παχυμερής, which means the substance of altered black bile consists of thick parts. This is the opposite of the description of vinegar, where Galen uses the term λεπτομερής, which means consisting of small parts. Elsewhere, we find that Galen asserts that substances consisting of thick parts are not able to react as much as those with small parts. One example, from *On Uneven Distemper*, compares yellow bile to black bile; the former is made of small parts and is easily changed by things it comes into contact with, while the latter, made of thicker parts is not so easily changed.[5] This type of language that refers to large and small parts is not found in the Hippocratic Corpus, but the notion of the difference in viscosity of the four humours implies that the density of the fluids affects their ability to flow freely through the body. We also

---

3 *At. Bil.* 4, CMG V 4,1,1, pp. 76,29–77,1 De Boer (V 115,10–14 K).

4 ἀλλ' εἰ καὶ κατὰ τοῦτο ἔοικεν ὄξει δριμυτάτῳ, τῷ παχυμερεῖ τῆς οὐσίας ἐναντιώτατα διάκειται καὶ διὰ τοῦτο, οἷς ἂν ὁμιλήσῃ τοῦ σώματος μέρεσιν ἄκρατος, ἑλκοῖ πάντως αὐτὰ διαβιβρώσκουσα. τὸ μὲν γὰρ ὄξος, ἅτε λεπτομερὲς ὄν, διεξέρχεται, τὸ δὲ τῆς μελαίνης χολῆς πάχος ἕδραν μόνιμον αὐτῇ παρέχον αἴτιον τῆς ἀναβρώσεως γίνεται. *At. Bil.* 3, CMG V 4,1,1, pp. 74,23–75,1 De Boer (V 111,6–12 K), adapted from a translation by Grant.

5 *Inaeq. Int.* III (VII 741,4–10 K), see also *Symp. Caus.* VI.4 (VII 119,5–16 K).

can find some comparable examples in the pseudo-Aristotelian *Problemata*. There is a passage in this text, which tells us that headaches in the morning are worse when wine is mixed, as unmixed wine contains thick parts, which cannot travel as far as mixed wine.[6] This is a similar to the way that Galen defines black bile as containing thick parts. The comparison between these two texts is further strengthened by the use of the same term ἄκρατος, which Galen uses to describe the pure black bile and the author of the passage from the *Problemata* uses for unmixed wine. We also find the use of the term λεπτομερής in another section of this text, where there is an explanation of substances that can sting the outside of the body and others the inside. This describes olive oil as having the smallest particles (λεπτομερέστατον), but in the next sentence names vinegar as the medicine of the flesh. By implication, vinegar too must contain small particles, which can pass through the loose texture of the flesh inside the body.[7] It is not certain that Galen is directly influenced by some of the passages from *Problemata* for his characterisation of the altered black bile by the size of particles and in relation to his comparison with vinegar. However, this type of language is not used by the authors of the extant Hippocratic Corpus, but it is used by later writers, such as the author of *Problemata* in the early Hellenistic period. This is an important part of Galen's characterisation of altered black bile, as it provides a mechanism to differentiate this state of the humour from similar acidic substances, such as vinegar.

We have seen from the two passages quoted from *On Black Bile* above (pages 94 and 96) that some of the most important characteristics of altered black bile are its sourness (στρυφνότητος), acidity (ὀξύτητος) and its ability to produce effervescence (ζυμοῖ). In fact, we have seen a similar description of altered black bile by Galen in the long section from *On the Natural Faculties* that I quoted above (page 79). The particular part that is important is '... because it also becomes acidic like vinegar and corrodes the animal's body, and the ground, if it be poured out upon it, and it produces a kind of fermentation and seething, accompanied by bubbles, ...'[8] Starting with the description of altered black bile based on the property of acidity, there are references to this humour

---

6 Pseudo-Aristotle, *Pr.* III.14, 873a5–8. Thomas' analysis suggests that a large amount of material in the *Problemata* is drawn from the Hippocratic Corpus, particularly from *Airs, Waters and Places, On Regimen II* and *Epidemics VI*. There are also some influences from *On the Sacred Disease, On Breaths, On Diseases I, II* and *III, Aphorisms* (section 6) and *On Affections*. See Thomas, 2015: 95–96.

7 Pseudo-Aristotle, *Pr.* XXXI.21, 959b5–14.

8 ... ὅτι καὶ δριμὺς ὁμοίως ὄξει γίγνεται καὶ ξύει γε τὸ σῶμα τοῦ ζῴου καὶ τὴν γῆν, εἰ κατ' αὐτῆς ἐκχυθείη, καί τινα μετὰ πομφολύγων οἷον ζύμωσίν τε καὶ ζέσιν ἐργάζεται ... *Nat. Fac.* II.9 (II 135,20–136,4 K), adapted from a translation by Brock.

being acidic (ὀξύς) in Galen's *Commentary on On the Nature of Man* and *On the Utility of the Parts*. However, in both of these texts there is no reference to the effervescent effect of altered black bile when in contact with earth.[9] But we do find this characteristic of effervescence elsewhere in Galen's writing. For example, we can find references to the 'bubbling' effect of altered black bile in some of his other works, such as *On the Therapeutic Method, Commentary on On Regimen in Acute Diseases* and *Commentary on Aphorisms*.[10] This is not the type of black bile that is described in the Hippocratic *On the Nature of Man*, but we do find that there are some comparable examples in other Hippocratic treatises.

The Hippocratic Corpus does not contain many references to substances having the properties of an acid in a similar way to how Galen describes altered black bile. However, we can find passages where there are some examples of these properties being exhibited by certain types of substance. For example, in the Hippocratic *On Regimen in Acute Diseases*, there is the following comparison between black bile and yellow (bitter) bile:

> It is said in summary, the acids from vinegar benefit those who suffer from bitter bile more than those who suffer from black bile. For the bitter humours are dissolved and turned into phlegm by it, not being brought up; but the black humours are fermented, brought up and multiplied, vinegar being apt to raise black humours. Vinegar on the whole is more harmful to women than men, for it is a cause of pain in the womb.[11]

This passage contains some important information for understanding Galen's writing on black bile. There is an association between black bile and fermen-

---

9   *HNH*, I.32, CMG V 9,1, p. 42,21–23 Mewaldt (XV 80,8–10 K). There is another example of this description in Galen's *UP* (V.4 (III 361,13–14 K)), where black bile is described as being sour (στρυφνή) and sharp (ὀξεῖα).

10   See *MM*, XIV.9 (X 974,11–14 K); *HVA*, III.38, CMG 9,1, p. 251.11–16 Helmreich (XV 693,6–12 K); *Hipp. Aph.* IV.24 (XVIIb 688,5–14 K).

11   Ἐν κεφαλαίῳ δὲ εἰρῆσθαι, αἱ ἀπὸ ὄξεος ὀξύτητες πικροχόλοισι μᾶλλον ἢ μελαγχολικοῖσι συμφέρουσι· τὰ μὲν γὰρ πικρὰ διαλύεται καὶ ἐκφλεγματοῦται ὑπ' αὐτοῦ οὐ μετεωριζόμενα· τὰ δὲ μέλανα ζυμοῦται καὶ μετεωρίζεται καὶ πολλαπλασιοῦται· ἀναγωγὸν γὰρ μελάνων ὄξος. γυναιξὶ δὲ τὸ ἐπίπαν πολεμιώτερον ἢ ἀνδράσιν ὄξος· ὑστεραλγὲς γάρ ἐστιν. *Acut.*, LXI (16L) (II 356,8–358,6 L), adapted from a translation by Jones. After the initial sentence, we have the substances denoted as 'bitter' (πικρά) and 'black' (μέλας) without the use of the term for 'bile' (χολή). It is typical of the author of this treatise to use this terminology for yellow bile and black bile and in fact there is no reference to 'black bile' as μέλαινα χολή, instead we find just 'black' (μέλας) or 'melancholic' (μελαγχολικός). However, Galen believed that *On Regimen in Acute Diseases* was a genuine work by Hippocrates and so would have accepted that these terms relate to the black bile humour. See chapter 2, section 3 above.

tation (ζυμοῦται) and the effect of vinegar (ὄξος) on black bile. This is similar to Galen's description of altered black bile in both *On Black Bile* and *On the Natural Faculties*. However, Galen does not quote or reference this Hippocratic passage from *On Regimen in Acute Diseases* in either of these treatises. But he does refer to it in *On the Powers of Simple Drugs*, where he attributes this statement about the beneficial and harmful effects on people suffering from yellow bile and black bile respectively. In addition to this, there is a brief reference to this passage in Galen's *Commentary on On Regimen in Acute Diseases*, but this only mentions those suffering from black bile and does not include any further detail about the importance of fermentation or vinegar for our understanding of altered black bile.[12] This means that this passage from *On Regimen in Acute Diseases* has been acknowledged by Galen as being important for the overall understanding of how two humours, such as yellow bile and altered black bile, can act differently in the body. It is significant, as we find that this Hippocratic text is distinctly characterising black bile in relation to acidity and effervescence, which Galen emphasises as the particular properties of altered black bile in *On Black Bile* and *On the Natural Faculties*. Therefore, Galen is characterising altered black bile in a way that is consistent with what we find in this passage from *On Regimen in Acute Diseases*. This is a way that Galen can bring together information on black bile from two different texts in the Hippocratic Corpus, such as *On the Nature of Man* and *On Regimen in Acute Diseases*, which seem to be about two completely separate substances. However, for Galen, the two texts contain information that he can use for the two different states of black bile.

Another text from the Hippocratic Corpus, which contains some material relating to the types of black substance that have properties of acidity and effervescence, is *On Diseases II*. For example, the following passage contains this description of evacuated waste substances from the body:

> Black disease: he vomits up black material that is like the lees of wine, sometimes blood-like, sometimes acidic like vinegar, sometimes saliva and scum, sometimes yellow-green bile. When he vomits up black blood-like material, it seems to smell of gore, his throat and mouth are burned by the vomitus, his teeth are set on edge, and the vomit raises the ground.[13]

---

12   *SMT*, I.33 (XI 438,12–14 K); *HVA*, III.61 CMG V 9,1 pp. 269,22–270,7 Helmreich (XV 730,17–731,16 K)). See Anastassiou and Irmer, 1997, volume II.1, pp. 3–4.

13   Μέλαινα· μέλαν ἐμέει οἷον τρύγα, τοτὲ δὲ αἱματῶδες, τοτὲ δὲ δριμὺ οἷον ὄξος, τοτὲ δὲ σίαλον καὶ λάπτην, τοτὲ δὲ χολὴν χλωρήν. καὶ ὅταν μὲν μέλαν καὶ τὸ αἱματῶδες ἐμέῃ, δοκέει οἷον φόνου ὄζειν, καὶ ἡ φάρυγξ καὶ τὸ στόμα καίεται ὑπὸ τοῦ ἐμέσματος, καὶ τοὺς ὀδόντας αἱμωδιᾷ, καὶ τὸ ἔμεσμα τὴν γῆν αἴρει. *Morb. II*, LXXIII (VII 110,14–19 L), adapted from a translation by Potter.

This is the type of situation that Galen was concerned about, where it is important to identify harmful substances, such as the altered black bile, within a mixture of waste matter. The first thing to note here is that this Hippocratic writer of *On Diseases II* does not refer to black bile explicitly in this passage. In fact, black bile is only directly referred to once in this whole treatise.[14] We have seen already that it seems that Galen had doubted the Hippocratic authenticity of this treatise.[15] However, it is possible that Galen may have ignored his rejection of *On Diseases II* as a Hippocratic text in order to make use of this type of harmful black substance that is similar to the way that he describes altered black bile. We can find a reference to a 'black disease', which Galen associated with black bile in his *Glossary of Hippocratic Terms*:

Black disease: the disease itself is said to be produced by black bile.[16]

It should be noted that this is the only reference that can be found in the extant Galenic Corpus that provides evidence that Galen may have used this section from *On Diseases II*, as if it were part of the authentic Hippocratic writing. Even though the link with Galen's glossary is dependent upon the textual similarity, I believe that there is reason to accept that Galen is naming the black substance in *On Diseases II* as black bile in his glossary.[17] This is because the vomited substances, produced when a person is suffering from the 'black disease', can be considered to share the most important characteristics with Galen's altered black bile. For example, we have some part of the evacuated substances being described as being acidic like vinegar (δριμὺ οἷον ὄξος), which we have seen in Galen's characterisation of altered black bile in treatises such as *On Black Bile* and *On the Natural Faculties*. Alongside this, we have the phrase 'the vomit raises the ground' (τὸ ἔμεσμα τὴν γῆν αἴρει), which Potter interprets as being the same meaning as 'causing the earth to froth and bubble'.[18] Combining these two properties of acidity of vinegar and causing the ground to 'bubble' means that this description of part of the substance described in *On*

---

14   *Morb. II*, VI (VII 14,11 L).
15   See chapter 2, section 3 above.
16   μέλαινα· λέγεται καὶ νόσος οὕτως ἀπὸ μελαίνης χολῆς συνισταμένη. *Gloss.* XIX 120,11–12 K.
17   Here I am following the research by Anastassiou and Irmer, who have linked this section of *On Diseases II* to Galen's definition in his *Glossary of Hippocratic Terms*. Further to this, there are more references to other parts of *On Diseases II* in Galen's glossary and he even names this treatise in some cases: *Gloss.* XIX 82,14–17; 84,16–17; 85,1–2; 89,16–18; 115,5–6; 121,12–14 K. For more examples see Anastassiou and Irmer, 1997, volume II.1, pp. 331–338.
18   Potter, 1988a: 329 (note 1).

Diseases II matches closely with Galen's characterisation of altered black bile. So even if Galen is not referring to this treatise in his glossary, it is possible that the description in this treatise may have had some influence on his writing on black bile.

If we look at other works from the Hippocratic Corpus, we can find that acidity is commonly used to explain the way that substances can cause great harm to the body. For example, in *Ancient Medicine* there is a passage relating to the effects of acid in the body:

> And those who are attacked by pungent and acrid acids suffer greatly from frenzy, from gnawing of the bowels and chest, and from restlessness. No relief from these symptoms is secured until the acidity is purged away, or calmed down and mixed with the other humours.[19]

The reference here to pungent (δριμύς) and acrid (ἰώδης) acids (ὀξύτης) is similar to what we found in *On Regimen in Acute Diseases*, *On Diseases II* and Galen's *On the Natural Faculties* and *On Black Bile*, which are related to the harmful effects of altered black bile. In addition, the use of the phrase 'gnaw at the bowels' (δήξιες σπλάγχνων) is also used by Galen when referring to the way that altered black bile can affect the body.[20] This shows that the very harmful effects of acidic substances in the body are important for doctors to understand the cause of severe disease so that they can provide the correct treatment. Galen does not quote or refer to the material in this passage from *Ancient Medicine* and we have seen that he has rejected the Hippocratic authenticity of this treatise.[21] However, it does show that the mechanism for damage to the intestines by acidic substances in the body was already part of medical theory at an early stage.

There is another text from the Hippocratic Corpus, *On Breaths*, which also describes the harmful effects of acidic substances:

> ... for phlegm, mixed with acrid humours produces sores wherever it strikes an unusual spot, and the throat, being soft, is roughened when a

---

19   καὶ ὅσοισι δὲ ὀξύτητες προσίστανται δριμεῖαί τε καὶ ἰώδεες, οἷαι λύσσαι καὶ δήξιες σπλάγχνων καὶ θώρηκος καὶ ἀπορίη· οὐ παύεταί τι τούτου πρότερον, πρὶν ἢ ἀποκαθαρθῇ τε καὶ καταστορεσθῇ καὶ μιχθῇ τοῖσιν ἄλλοισιν· VM, XIX (I 618,6–15 L), translation by Jones.

20   In *At. Bil.* (5, CMG V 4,1,1, p. 80,7–15 De Boer (V 122,2–123,3 K)), we are told that both yellow bile and black bile can eat away (διαβιβρώσκω) at the intestines (ἔντερον).

21   See chapter 2, section 3 above.

flux strikes it ... Being acrid the phlegm ulcerates the flesh when it strikes it, and bursts open the veins.[22]

Here again we have a description of the harmful effects of acidic substances on the body. This time the emphasis is on phlegm, which the author of *On Breaths* tells us is either mixed with (unnamed) acrid humours (δριμέσι χυμοῖσι μεμιγμένον) or is an acidic (δριμὺ) substance itself. In contrast, to the author of *On Breaths*, Galen has associated this type of ulceration with the harmful effect of altered black bile rather than with phlegm.[23] There is also a type of 'acidic phlegm' described in Plato's *Timaeus*, which is a mixture of blood and acidic bile and has some saline properties.[24] Therefore, there does seem to be a development of a harmful type of phlegm, which has acidic properties in the early work on medical issues presented in *On Breaths* and possibly in Plato's *Timaeus*. This indicates that there was a tradition in medical writing to explain potentially harmful substances in the body based on the acidic properties of humours, such as bile and phlegm. Galen continues this tradition by assigning a particular state of black bile with acidity that is dangerous because it is harmful to the body. This goes far beyond the black bile described in the Hippocratic *On the Nature of Man*, as Galen, from the point of view of other Hippocratic works and the medical writing of other authorities, needs to include this type of characterisation of black bile in his biological model.

2   Summary

We have seen that Galen's construction of a biological theory based on different types of black bile contains a description of a form of black bile that is very harmful to the body. We have found that Galen describes this type of black bile as having very acidic properties and tells us that it effervesces when it comes into contact with the ground. It is very important for Galen that altered black bile can be correctly and consistently identified in the waste material evacuated from the body, in order for doctors to be able to make good diagnoses and

---

22   ... τὸ γὰρ φλέγμα δριμέσι χυμοῖσι μεμιγμένον, ὅπη ἂν προσπέσῃ ἐς ἀήθεας τόπους, ἑλκοῖ· τῇ δὲ φάρυγγι ἁπαλῇ ἐούσῃ ῥεῦμα προσπῖπτον τρηχύτητας ἐμποιεῖ· ... δριμὺ δὲ ἐὸν τὸ φλέγμα προσ-πῖπτόν τε τῇ σαρκὶ ἑλκοῖ καὶ ἀναρρηγνύει τὰς φλέβας. *Flat.* VII; VIII; X (VI 100,10–12; 21–22; 106,3–6; 14–15 L), translation by Jones.

23   *At. Bil.* 3, CMG V 4,1,1, pp. 74,23–75,1 De Boer (V 111,6–12 K) and Galen, *UP*, V.10 (III 381,6–382,5 K).

24   Plato, *Tim.*, 83c–d.

prognoses. In *On Regimen in Acute Diseases*, we find that black bile is explicitly referred to in relation to the acidic properties of vinegar. This is a treatise that Galen considered to be Hippocratic and so it is a good source for him to show that Hippocrates is in agreement with the existence of this altered form of black bile. However, in *On Diseases II*, we have the characterisation of a substance that is acidic and even reacts with the ground in a similar way to Galen's description of altered black bile. It is possible that Galen has referenced this passage in his *Glossary of Hippocratic Terms* when he associates its content with black bile. If this is the case, then Galen has acknowledged a passage from *On Diseases II* as being consistent with Hippocratic doctrine and so he is able to draw upon it for his own characterisation of black bile, as if it were part of one of the texts that he considers to be Hippocratic. This goes far beyond the ideas contained in the Hippocratic *On the Nature of Man* and shows that Galen is attempting to reconcile his observations with what he considers to be authentic Hippocratic doctrine. Therefore, if we want to understand why Galen is presenting black bile in a particular way, then we need to know the context of the treatise. This allows us to avoid the problems associated with trying to make Galen's characterisation of black bile fit into some theoretical system that somehow has to be consistent with different Galenic treatises and the Hippocratic *On the Nature of Man*.

CHAPTER 6

The Cleansing of Harmful Black Bile from the Body

In this chapter I will investigate Galen's theory of how the different types of black bile are produced and managed in the body. Galen provides much more information on the removal of black bile than on its generation in the body. Therefore, there will be more analysis on the way that Galen describes the spleen as the organ that attracts and removes 'black bile' from the body. We shall see that Galen's explanation of the management of black bile depends on the context of his writing in a particular treatise. However, before investigating Galen's writing on the spleen and black bile, it is worthwhile considering his view on how black bile is generated in the body and for this we must start with the liver.

1   The Importance of the Liver for the Origin of Black Bile in the Body

The liver is the organ that is most generally associated with the generation of yellow bile and black bile in the body, which can be found in some of Galen's treatises.[1] The evidence for the production of yellow bile in the liver can be found in Galen's *On the Utility of the Parts*, as there is a mechanism that allows for the separation of yellow bile from blood by vessels in the liver that connect to the gallbladder.[2] However, when it comes to black bile, the situation is more complex because, as we have seen above, Galen differentiates between different types of black bile. For example, in *On the Utility of the Parts*, Galen tells us that the spleen removes the 'muddy, thick, melancholic humours formed in the liver' (τῶν ἐν ἥπατι γεννωμένων ἰλυωδῶν καὶ παχέων καὶ μελαγχολικῶν χυμῶν), which is the type that I have named non-ideal natural black bile, as opposed to the ideal natural or altered types of black bile.[3] It is interesting that Galen uses the plural term 'melancholic humours' (μελαγχολικοὶ χυμοί) in this passage, as he tends to use the singular for this term more often in his writing.[4]

---

1   Arikha, 2007: 26–27.
2   *UP*, IV.13 (III 306,11–13 K).
3   *UP*, IV.15 (III 316,13–17 K), translation by May. See Siegel, 1968: 260–261; 270.
4   There are a few other examples when he uses the plural: for example in *At. Bil.* (8, CMG V 4,1,1, p. 91,22–24 De Boer (V 143,15–144,2 K)), where Galen uses this plural form once in a statement about how some people are confused by distinctions between melancholic humours.

This suggests that he wants to emphasise the production of different types of non-ideal natural black bile in the liver under these conditions. We have seen already that Galen also uses the term 'melancholic humour' to refer to different types of altered black bile.[5] However, I think that it is likely that only forms of non-ideal natural black bile are present in the liver under normal conditions, as altered black bile is produced by the extreme heating of natural black bile, yellow bile or blood in any part of the body. We can find more evidence for the association between the liver and black bile from a passage in *On Affected Parts*, where we are told that: '[the spleen] draws the melancholic blood from the liver to itself, ...'.[6] In this passage Galen is using the term 'melancholic blood' to refer to a type of non-ideal natural black bile that is drawn out of the liver to the spleen. This is part of the process in the body that ensures that the blood has the correct balance of the essential qualities and only requires a small amount of black bile to thicken the blood and add the paired quantities of 'cold and dry' to the overall humoral mixture in the blood. Galen has chosen to refer to the non-ideal natural black bile as 'melancholic blood' perhaps indicating that the spleen draws out the 'thick, cold and dry' substances from the liver, rather than the actual ideal natural black bile, which is the innate humour and is required for health. This is supported by a brief statement in *On Affected Parts* where we are told that the ideal natural black bile is generated in the blood vessels from certain foodstuffs.[7]

The process of adding small quantities of the natural forms of black bile is finely balanced, as excess amounts of natural black bile can cause harm in the body. This is shown in the following passage from *On the Natural Faculties*:

> There is, however, a natural use for the humours first mentioned, both thick and thin; the blood is purified both by the spleen and by the bladder beside the liver, and a part of each of the two humours is put away, of such quantity and quality that, if it were carried all over the body of the animal, it would do a certain amount of harm. For that which is sufficiently thick and earth-like, and has entirely escaped alteration in the liver, the spleen draws into itself; the other part, which is moderately thick, having been pressed hard alongside the other, is carried all over the body. For the blood in many parts of the animal needs, I believe a certain amount of thickening, as does the fibrin carried within it.[8]

---

5 See chapter 4, section 1 above.
6 τὸ μελαγχολικὸν ἐκ τοῦ ἥπατος ἕλκειν αἷμα εἰς ἑαυτὸν, ... *Loc. Aff.* VI.1 (VIII 377,10–378,1 K).
7 *Loc. Aff.* III.9 (VIII 177,9–12 K), see chapter 4, section 1 above.
8 τῶν δ' εἰρημένων χυμῶν ἐστί τις χρεία τῇ φύσει καὶ τοῦ παχέος καὶ τοῦ λεπτοῦ καὶ καθαίρεται πρός

The 'humours' at the beginning of this passage are the different types of bile, which include the various forms of black bile, both natural and altered. However, Galen makes particular reference to the bile that is 'thick' (παχύς) and 'earth-like' (γεώδης), which is the way he characterises natural black bile.[9] Galen is pointing out that the body requires a mechanism to purify the blood; otherwise the proper balance of the qualities in the humoral mixture cannot be maintained.

We can see from this passage that in Galen's theory of the body, a certain amount of black bile is required. This is the ideal form of black bile and the system Galen describes here helps to maintain the balance of this humour. The type of black bile drawn to the spleen is the non-ideal black bile, just as we saw in the passage from *On Affected Parts* above. This means that we must ingest the correct amount of certain food and drink to produce enough black bile in the body and any excess will cause the blood to be thicker and can be reduced by the spleen. The liver appears to be a point in the body where this thick, cold and dry substance either is drawn into the blood for nourishment, or is taken up by the spleen so that it can be removed from the body. If the black bile is in the optimum state of coldness, dryness and thickness, then it is ideal, otherwise it is considered to be non-ideal and must be removed from the body in order to avoid the diseases associated with an excess of this humour.[10] When Galen uses the terms 'black bile' (μέλαινα χολή) and 'melancholic humour' (μελαγχολικὸς χυμός) interchangeably, it can be difficult to ascertain the specific state of black bile at various points in the body, such as its movement between the blood vessels, liver and spleen. Galen tends to use melancholic humour or melancholic blood for the non-ideal type of black bile. However, we have already seen that the melancholic humours have the potential to become either ideal natural

---

τε τοῦ σπληνὸς καὶ τῆς ἐπὶ τῷ ἥπατι κύστεως τὸ αἷμα καὶ ἀποτίθεται τοσοῦτόν τε καὶ τοιοῦτον ἑκατέρου μέρος, ὅσον καὶ οἷον, εἴπεο εἰς ὅλον ἠνέχθη τοῦ ζῴου τὸ σῶμα, βλάβην ἄν τιν' εἰργάσατο. τὸ γὰρ ἱκανῶς παχὺ καὶ γεῶδες καὶ τελέως διαπεφευγὸς τὴν ἐν τῷ ἥπατι μεταβολὴν ὁ σπλὴν εἰς ἑαυτὸν ἕλκει· τὸ δ' ἄλλο τὸ μετρίως παχὺ σὺν τῷ κατειργάσθαι πάντη φέρεται. δεῖται γὰρ ἐν πολ-λοῖς τοῦ ζῴου μορίοις παχύτητός τινος τὸ αἷμα καθάπερ οἶμαι καὶ τῶν ἐμφερομένων ἰνῶν. *Nat. Fac.* II.9 (II 138,7–139,1 K), adapted from a translation by Brock.

9   See chapter 3, section 1 above.

10   I cannot find any references to this type of information on the generation of black bile in the body in the Hippocratic Corpus, or the writing of the other physicians such as Diocles and Rufus of Ephesus. But in Aristotle's *Parts of Animals*, we are told that the earthy (γεώ-δης) fibrin causes the blood to congeal when the more fluid part is evaporated. In Plato's *Timaeus* the fibrin is described as viscid (γλίσχρος) and oily (λιπαρός). Aristotle, *PA*, II.4, 650b15–19; Plato, *Tim.* 82c–d. See LS&J, page 836.

black bile or altered black bile if they remain in the body.[11] When it comes to the health of the body, we can see that in Galen's system black bile is able to nourish the blood and many different parts of the body, as it has the required qualities of thickness, dryness and coldness. However, there are not many references to this process, even in Galen's treatises, which might indicate that he did not consider this a topic requiring detailed explanation in his writing on black bile.

2 The Relationship between the Structure of the Spleen and Its Function

We have seen above that for Galen the spleen is the organ that is most strongly associated with the overall management and removal of black bile in the body. Galen provides information about the structure and function of the spleen in *On the Utility of the Parts*:

> But now let us inspect the remaining features in the construction of the spleen and first of all its particular feature, which some call the parenchyma. This is what gives the spleen the faculty of attracting the melancholic humours; it is extremely loose textured and porous like a sponge to enable it easily to attract and receive the thickness of these humours.[12]

This passage tells us that the spleen's structure is important, as it is designed to attract and accommodate the thick humours. We can see that Galen draws our attention to the importance of the 'parenchyma' (παρέγχυμα), which in *On Mixtures* he attributes to the Erasistrateans.[13] This substance gives the spleen the properties of being 'extremely loose textured' (ἀραιὸν ἱκανῶς) and porous

---

11 We have seen that Galen uses the term οὐδέπω 'not yet' in reference to the potential of melancholic humour to become the ideal type of black bile. See chapter 4, section 1 above.

12 ἀλλὰ νῦν γε τὰ ὑπόλοιπα τῆς κατασκευῆς τοῦ σπληνὸς ἐπισκεψώμεθα καὶ πρῶτον τὸ ἴδιον αὐτοῦ σῶμα τὸ καλούμενον ὑπό τινων παρέγχυμα. τοῦτ' οὖν ἐστιν αὐτό, καθ' ὃ τοὺς μελαγχολικοὺς ἕλκειν εἰς ἑαυτὸν ὁ σπλὴν δύναμιν ἔχει χυμούς, ἀραιὸν ἱκανῶς καὶ χαῦνον ὑπάρχον ὥσπερ τις σπογγιὰ πρὸς τὸ ῥᾳδίως ἕλκειν τε καὶ παραδέχεσθαι τὸ πάχος αὐτῶν. *UP*, IV.15 (III 318,1–7 K), adapted from a translation by May.

13 The Erasistrateans described the lungs, liver, kidneys and spleen as appearing to be 'poured beside' (παρέγχυμα) the veins that are attached to them. For example, *Temp.* II.3 (II 599,16–600,4 K); *AA*, VI.11; VII.5 (II 576,12–19; 603,5–7); cf. Pseudo-Galen, *Int.*, IX (XIV 697,8–698,1 K). See LS&J page 1332; Leith, 2015b: 253–255.

(χαῦνον), in this way the spleen is said to be 'like a sponge' (ὥσπερ τις σπογγιά).[14] There is a treatise in the Hippocratic Corpus, which provides similar physiological detail about the role of the spleen as an organ that cleanses harmful substances in the body. We find in *On Diseases IV* a theory of four 'moistures' in the body, blood, phlegm, bile and the watery fluid, the last of which is associated with the spleen that is its 'spring'. This 'spring' is described as being hollow, like the head, and has an attractive power that specifically draws in this watery fluid. This Hippocratic author uses the term 'attract' (ἕλκω) for the way that the spleen can bring the watery fluid to itself. Also, like the case of the spleen and black bile, the excess watery fluid that is brought to the spleen must then go to the bladder to be passed out of the body. Failure to do this will result in pain and ultimately disease in the spleen.[15] However, Galen did not acknowledge the Hippocratic authenticity of *On Diseases IV* and he does not mention this text at all in any of his extant treatises. We would expect Galen to reject this theory on the basis that it refers to the watery fluid, rather than black bile, as in *On the Utility of the Parts* Galen explains that the larger vessels leading to the spleen are specifically designed to transport a thicker liquid, such as non-ideal natural black bile.

The passage from *On the Utility of the Parts* above also provides information on the type of substance that the spleen attracts from the blood. The reference to thick melancholic humours indicates that these are the non-ideal forms of natural black bile. Just before this passage, Galen tells us that there are arteries, which are the location for the transformation of different types of non-ideal natural bile from certain nutrients that have been ingested into the body. These arteries provide continuous motion (τῷ διηνεκεῖ τῆς κινήσεως) and strength of innate heat (τῇ τῆς ἐμφύτου θερμασίας ἰσχύι) that comes from the heart. This allows non-ideal natural black bile to be prepared for use (κατεργάζομαι), broken up (καταθραύω) and changed (μεταβάλλω).[16] This could indicate that the non-ideal natural black bile is being prepared for its useful role as part of the humoral mixture, essential for the health of the body. Alternatively, any excess and unwanted non-ideal natural black bile can be either broken up for removal from the body or possibly changed into something else, although Galen does

---

14　However, Galen's use of the term parenchyma is different from the Erasistratean concept of this type of substance, as they believed that it served as structural material supporting the *Triplokia* of arteries, veins and nerves. See Leith, 2015b: 251–262.

15　*Morb. IV,* II (33 L); VI (37L); IX (40 L); XXVI (57 L), (VII 542,18–544,21; 552,20–554,15; 560,7–562,5; 610,1–614,4 L).

16　*UP,* IV.15 (III 316,17–317,11 K). We have seen in *On Black Bile* that Galen describes a type of non-ideal natural black bile drawn into the spleen from the blood as similar to the watery part of olive oil. But this would still be much thicker than the watery fluid of *On Diseases IV.*

not elaborate any further on this process of transformation. Another example, this time from *On Black Bile*, tells us more about the substance that is drawn to the spleen:

> Swayed, therefore, by these things, the best of the doctors and philosophers of the past spoke out that the liver is cleansed by the spleen, which drew into itself what is muddy in the blood. Such things are, as I was saying, like the lees in wine or the watery part of olive oil.[17]

In this passage we find a substance that is characterised by the terms 'muddy' (ἰλυῶδες) and 'lees in wine' (ἐν οἴνῳ μὲν ἡ τρύξ), which we have seen are associated with non-ideal natural black bile.[18] In *On the Therapeutic Method*, we are told that the spleen removes much of the material that is mud-like (ἰλυῶδες), which is related to the melancholic humour (μελαγχολικὸς χυμός), from the liver and again this is a familiar description of non-ideal natural black bile.[19] Galen makes a similar statement in *On the Causes of Symptoms*, where we are told that the blood is purified of yellow bile and serum by the gallbladder and kidneys respectively, and 'the spleen purifies the blood of the melancholic humour' (ἐκκαθαίρει τὸ μελαγχολικὸν ὁ σπλήν).[20] Galen sometimes uses more descriptive language, as we find in *On the Formation of the Foetus*, where he refers to some types of non-ideal natural black bile as the 'muddy residues' (ἰλυώδη περιττώματα), which are cleansed by the spleen.[21] In *On Black Bile*, there are two passages where Galen refers to the μελαγχολικὸς χυμός being attracted to the spleen from the blood. But in one case, Galen uses the term μέλαινα χολή, rather than μελαγχολικὸς χυμός in association with the spleen.[22] There is also a passage in *Commentary on Epidemics* where Galen uses the term μέλαινα χολή in relation to the spleen.[23] We can also find references to a μελαγχολικὸς χυμός and the

---

17 διὰ τούτων μὲν οὖν ὑπαχθέντες οἱ ἄριστοι τῶν παλαιῶν ἰατρῶν τε καὶ φιλοσόφων ἀπεφήναντο καθαίρεσθαι τὸ ἧπαρ ὑπὸ τοῦ σπληνός, ἕλκοντος εἰς ἑαυτὸν ὅσον ἰλυῶδες ἐν αἵματι. τοιοῦτον δὲ τοῦτό ἐστιν, ὡς ἔφην, ὁποῖον ἐν οἴνῳ μὲν ἡ τρύξ, ἐν ἐλαίῳ δὲ ἀμόργη. At. Bil. 6, CMG V 4,1,1, p. 83,11–14 De Boer (V 127,12–17 K), adapted from a translation by Grant.

18 Galen also brings in another characterisation, saying that the substance is similar to the 'watery part of olive oil'. This comparison to olive oil is not a common description used by Galen, but it is found in MM (XIV.9 (X 975,1–6 K)) as well to describe black bile.

19 MM, XIII.17 (X 920,7–10 K).

20 Symp. Caus. III.2 (VII 222,10–14 K). See Siegel, 1968: 271.

21 Foet. Form. V (IV 686,2–3 K).

22 At. Bil. 7–9, CMG V 4,1,1, pp. 87,15–16; 89,15–18; 93,16–19 De Boer (V 136,1–3; 139,17–140,2; 147,3–7 K).

23 Hipp. Epid. VI.V.14 CMG V 10,2,2, p. 286,17–18 Wenkebach (XVIIb 274,7–8 K).

spleen in Galen's *Commentary on Epidemics* and *Commentary on Aphorisms*.[24]
Therefore, when he is describing the substance that is removed from the blood
by the spleen, Galen often uses the term 'melancholic humour' (μελαγχολικὸς
χυμός). This implies that the function of the spleen is to attract and remove the
non-ideal natural black bile, which is the thicker, colder, or drier type of black
bile such as the sediment, muddy or lees-like substances that characterise this
form of black bile. In these cases where Galen talks about the function of the
spleen he does not refer to the other types of black bile. The reason for this may
be that the ideal form of natural black bile is used by Galen when referring to
the normal, healthy state of the body and so does not need to be removed from
the humoral mixture with the other humours in the composite blood. If ideal
natural black bile becomes excessive and has to be removed, then it is possible
that Galen would classify it as a 'melancholic humour' (μελαγχολικὸς χυμός),
as it might be observed because of its thickening of the blood and could form
a precipitate that is associated with his description of the non-ideal forms of
natural black bile.

Further to this, we can find information on the function of the spleen in
On the Natural Faculties. Here we find Galen discussing the situation when the
spleen is not functioning properly:

> For in general, whenever [the spleen] is drawing the melancholic humour
> into itself to a much lesser amount than is fitting, the blood is unpurged,
> the whole body takes on a bad colour. When does [the spleen] draw in
> to a much lesser amount? Clearly because it is in a bad condition. Then,
> just as the kidneys, whose function it is to attract the urine, do this badly
> when they are out of order, so with the spleen, having the capacity in itself
> of attracting the melancholic quality, when this natural attraction devel-
> ops a weakness, it must attract badly and in the process the blood must
> become immediately thicker and blacker.[25]

In this passage Galen uses μελαγχολικὸς χυμός, which is the only place in this
treatise where he refers to this specific term. This supports the view that Galen

---

24   *Hipp. Epid.* VI.II.44, CMG V 10,2,2, p. 115,10–12 Wenkebach (XVIIa 994,12–14 K); *Hipp. Aph.*
       III.22; IV.21 (XVIIb 622,6–9; 682,3–5 K); VI.43 (XVIIIa 67,7–9 K).
25   καθόλου γάρ, ὅταν ἐνδεέστερον ἢ προσῆκεν εἰς ἑαυτὸν ἕλκῃ τὸν μελαγχολικὸν χυμόν, ἀκάθαρτον
       μὲν τὸ αἷμα, κακόχρουν δὲ τὸ πᾶν γίγνεται σῶμα. πότε δ' ἐνδεέστερον ἕλκει; ἢ δῆλον ὅτι κακῶς
       διακείμενος. ὥσπερ οὖν τοῖς νεφροῖς ἐνεργείας οὔσης ἕλκειν τὰ οὖρα κακῶς ἕλκειν ὑπάρχει κακο-
       πραγοῦσιν, οὕτω καὶ τῷ σπληνὶ ποιότητος μελαγχολικῆς ἑλκτικὴν ἐν ἑαυτῷ δύναμιν ἔχοντι σύμ-
       φυτον ἀρρωστήσαντί ποτε ταύτην ἀναγκαῖον ἕλκειν κακῶς κἂν τῷδε παχύτερον ἤδη καὶ μελάν-
       τερον γίγνεσθαι τὸ αἷμα. *Nat. Fac.* II.9 (II 133,8–17 K), adapted from a translation by Brock.

explains the function of the spleen as being designed to remove non-ideal natural black bile from the blood, which is the type of melancholic humour that is thick and has the potential to become the ideal type of black bile if it remains in the body. This means that if the spleen is not working properly, then the blood becomes thicker and darker, indicating that too much black bile is present in the body. There is more evidence for this in another passage, from *On Black Bile*, where Galen tells us that the body can be observed to be discoloured, if the spleen becomes impaired in some way, and in this text he actually gives specific causes of its reduction in performance due to inflammation (φλεγμονή), induration (σκίρρος, a hardened swelling) or enervation (ἀτονία, a slackening).[26] So the spleen is designed to remove potentially harmful non-ideal black bile from the blood, but what about the even more dangerous altered black bile? We have seen in *On the Natural Faculties* and *On Black Bile* that Galen believes that the altered form of black bile has changed its innate qualities to become hot in potential and acidic in its corrosive effects on other substances. I think that Galen has postulated that the spleen fulfils a natural process in the body that is equivalent to the purgation of potentially harmful non-ideal natural black bile by a drug, such as hellebore, which draws out this humour. Therefore, the spleen was not designed to attract or cope with the altered form of black bile with its acidic and corrosive properties. This is why altered black bile is so dangerous, as the natural process of removal by the spleen is not designed to manage this substance. It is therefore important for Galen to provide advice on how to make a correct identification of the symptoms and observational evidence for the presence of altered black bile in the body and what intervention might remove this harmful substance from the body as quickly as possible.

We can compare Galen's description of the structure and function of the spleen with earlier sources, such as the following passage from Plato's *Timaeus*:

> On which account, whenever certain impurities, on account of bodily diseases, are produced around the liver, the loose texture of the spleen receives all these impurities and cleanses them, seeing that it is constructed of hollow and bloodless [material]. Whence being full of the waste matter, it grows large and festered by sores, and in contrast, whenever the body is cleansed, [the spleen] decreases in size, collapsing down into itself.[27]

---

26   *At. Bil.* 6, CMG V 4,1,1, p. 83,1–3 De Boer (V 126,18–127,3 K). I will be discussing diseases of the spleen in more detail later, see section 4 below.

27   διὸ δὴ καὶ ὅταν τινὲς ἀκαθαρσίαι γίγνωνται διὰ νόσους σώματος περὶ τὸ ἧπαρ, πάντα ἡ σπληνὸς καθαίρουσα αὐτὰ δέχεται μανότης, ἅτε κοίλου καὶ ἀναίμου ὑφανθέντος· ὅθεν πληρούμενος τῶν

If we start with Plato's description of the structure of the spleen, we find that he has characterised this organ as having a 'loose texture' (μανότης) and is hollow (κοῖλος) and bloodless (ἄναιμος). The structure explains the way that the spleen attracts and cleanses certain impurities in the body. This is similar to Galen's explanation of the way that the spleen attracts the non-ideal natural black bile in the passage from *On the Utility of the Parts* that I quoted earlier (see page 107 above). However, when it comes to the actual substance that is said to be drawn in and purged by the spleen, we find from this passage in Plato's *Timaeus* that he only refers to 'certain impurities' (τινὲς ἀκαθαρσίαι) produced by disease in the body. This is a more general description that explains the cleansing power of the spleen expressed in relation to anything pathogenic produced around the liver that needs removing from the body.[28] If we investigate the Hippocratic Corpus, it is more difficult to find this type of description of the structure of the spleen. One possible source is *Ancient Medicine*, which refers to the spongy (σπογγοειδέα) and porous (ἀραιά) structure of the spleen that allows it to easily draw in fluids. The author of *Ancient Medicine* is writing in a similar way to Galen to explain the function of an organ from its structural properties.[29] However, Galen was generally unimpressed with this treatise and did not regard it as a genuine Hippocratic work and he does not make any reference to this material on the spleen.[30] In another text from the Hippocratic Corpus, *On Fleshes*, we find a description of the structure of the spleen based on two fundamental substances, the fatty (λιπαρός) and the gluey (κολλώδης). These two substances form in just the right way from the action of heat to create the soft (μαλακός) and fibrous (ἰνῶδες) structure of the spleen.[31] However, there are no equivalent fundamental entities in Galen's writing to these fatty and gluey substances when he describes the fundamental structure of the parts of the body.[32] Therefore, we can see that there is similarity between Galen's structure of the spleen with what we find in earlier treatises, such as Plato's

---

ἀποκαθαιρομένων μέγας καὶ ὕπουλος αὐξάνεται, καὶ πάλιν, ὅταν καθαρθῇ τὸ σῶμα, ταπεινούμε-
νος εἰς ταὐτὸν ξυνίζει. Plato, *Tim.* 72c–d, adapted from a translation by Bury.

28   In addition to this passage in Plato's *Timaeus*, Aristotle (*PA*, III.7, 670b4–8) tells us that the spleen attracts excessive moisture (ἰκμάδας περιττευούσας) from the stomach.

29   *VM*, XXII (I 628,9–12 L). See Jouanna, 2001: 315.

30   See chapter 2, section 3 above.

31   *Carn.* III (VIII 584,19–588,13 L). See Jouanna, 2001: 279 and Nutton, 2004: 75.

32   In *PHP* (VIII.6.55, CMG V 4,1,2, p. 522,32–33 De Lacy (V 701,16–702,1 K)), Galen describes a waste product from the body as being similar to yellow bile, which is fatty. The term gluey is used throughout *On the Powers of Foodstuffs*, for example in one case (1.6, CMG V 4,2, p. 226,9–10 Helmreich (VI 497,8–9 K)), when describing the preparation of groats, which quickly thickens and congeals (κολλώδης).

Timaeus and the Hippocratic *Ancient Medicine*. But, we do not find any explicit reference to either of these passages in any of Galen's extant works when he is discussing the function of the spleen in relation to black bile. However, the closeness to Plato's description of the structure of the spleen allows Galen to claim that Plato is in agreement with him. But there is a discrepancy, as in other treatises such as *On the Utility of the Parts* and *On the Natural Faculties*, Galen specifically refers to the function of the spleen in relation to its management of non-ideal natural black bile in the body. But, as we shall see, Galen has certain polemical reasons to emphasise the function of the spleen for the specific attraction of black bile.

3   Galen's Attack on Asclepiades and Erasistratus on the Function of the Spleen to Cleanse the Body of Black Bile

There are specific reasons why Galen wanted to emphasise the function of the spleen in its role in the management of black bile. As we shall see, Galen reacts to what he perceives to be some consensus that black bile and the spleen are not important in medicine. In order to refute this opinion, Galen presents a number of arguments to defend his own view that knowledge of black bile and the spleen and the relationship between them, is of paramount importance for the best medical practice. I will start with Galen's criticism of Asclepiades in *On the Natural Faculties*:

> He (Asclepiades) also talks no less nonsense about black bile and the spleen, not understanding what was said by Hippocrates; and he attempts in stupid—I might say insane—language, to contradict what he knows nothing about.[33]

Firstly, we have already seen that Galen had a generally low opinion of Asclepiades' theory of medicine.[34] The context of the passage quoted above is Galen's general criticism of Asclepiades' corpuscular theory of elements, which he considers as inferior to his own theory of qualities, elements and humours. He also rejects what he presents as Asclepiades' theory of the generation of yellow bile in the bile-ducts and the idea that a person suffering from the disease

---

33   ληρεῖ δ᾽ οὐδὲν ἧττον καὶ περὶ τῆς μελαίνης χολῆς καὶ τοῦ σπληνὸς οὔτε τί ποθ᾽ ὑφ᾽ Ἱπποκράτους εἴρηται συνιεὶς ἀντιλέγειν τ᾽ ἐπιχειρῶν οἷς οὐκ οἶδεν ἐμπλήκτῳ τινὶ καὶ μανικῷ στόματι. *Nat. Fac.* I.13 (II 40,8–12 K), translation by Brock.
34   See chapter 2, section 4 above.

jaundice, can be full of yellow bile, but will not evacuate it. This seems to be in the same context as his criticism of Asclepiades' writing on black bile and the spleen.[35] Galen does not tell us exactly what Asclepiades said, but we can infer that Galen is accusing him of rejecting the notion that the spleen will attract black bile from the blood and remove it from the body. We know that Galen himself regarded the spleen as the organ that regulates the non-ideal natural black bile in the body, and in this passage he suggests that Hippocrates has this same opinion of the function of the spleen. One thing to note here is that Galen uses the term 'black bile' (μέλαινα χολή), rather than 'melancholic humour' (μελαγχολικὸς χυμός). This is an example of the interchangeability of these two terms. The reason that Galen chooses μέλαινα χολή here might be that it is a more general statement about Asclepiades' theory, and so Galen would want to refer to the more recognised term for 'black bile' as one of the four humours of the body. However, when he is providing detail about the physiology of black bile and the function of the humour, it might seem more correct to Galen to use μελαγχολικὸς χυμός. This is a situation where Galen is merging the different types of natural black bile, both the ideal and non-ideal forms, as it is more convenient for him to make a general statement about 'black bile' and the spleen when he is criticising a rival theory in this way. This is why it is important for Galen not to apply a restrictive system of nomenclature, as it would force him to use specific terms such as μελαγχολικὸς χυμός when he would prefer to use μέλαινα χολή or vice-versa. This is consistent with what we have seen already when Galen justifies 'looseness of language' because he claims that he has the proper knowledge of the different forms of black bile.

In another part of *On the Natural Faculties*, Galen makes a similar complaint against Erasistratus, and again refers to Hippocrates as an authority on the spleen and black bile:

> Has Erasistratus, then, not read the book, *On the Nature of Man*, any more than any of the rest of Hippocrates's writings, in order that he so lazily passes over the investigation of the humours, or having done this, purposely leaves on one side the most beautiful theories of the 'art' [of medicine]? Or, does he know it, and yet voluntarily neglect one of the finest studies in medicine? Thus he ought not to have said anything about the spleen, nor have stultified himself by holding that an artistic Nature would have prepared so large an organ for no purpose. As a matter of fact, not only Hippocrates and Plato—who are no less authorities on Nature

---

35   *Nat. Fac.* I.13 (II 39,4–40,8 K).

than is Erasistratus—say that this organ is one of those which cleanse the blood, but also thousands of others, both ancient physicians and philosophers, who are in agreement.[36]

From these two passages from *On the Natural Faculties*, we can see that Galen accuses both Asclepiades and Erasistratus of not following Hippocrates' theory of the humours. This is not only an issue concerning the humours, but is a broader problem for these physicians, as Galen asserts that they have moved away from what he considers the correct teleological theory of the body that he traces back to the work of Hippocrates and Aristotle.[37] However, I think that Galen goes further than this general teleological view, as he specifically emphasises Asclepiades' and Erasistratus' ignorance of what Hippocrates has said about the spleen and black bile. In the passage above, Galen also brings in Plato as an authority on the function of the spleen, along with many other ancient physicians and philosophers. We can see that Galen explicitly refers to *On the Nature of Man* in relation to the humours. But Galen also names Hippocrates as having said that the spleen is the organ that cleanses the blood. Galen's reference to *On the Nature of Man* at the beginning of this passage may suggest that this text is important for understanding the role of the spleen to manage black bile. However, there are only a couple of passages in this treatise that refer to this organ:

... under the breast both to the spleen and to the kidneys, ... and from the ribs above one [vein] reaches to the spleen and the other to the liver, ...[38]

This is the part of *On the Nature of Man* that presents the author's anatomical knowledge of how the various blood vessels connect to the major organs in the body. The spleen is part of these overall interconnections and therefore is

---

36 ἆρ᾽ οὖν οὔτε τῶν ἄλλων ἀνέγνω τι τῶν Ἱπποκράτους γραμμάτων Ἐρασίστρατος οὐδέν, οὔτε τὸ περὶ φύσεως ἀνθρώπου βιβλίον, ἵν᾽ οὕτως ἀργῶς παρέλθοι τὴν περὶ τῶν χυμῶν ἐπίσκεψιν, ἢ γιγνώσκει μέν, ἑκὼν δὲ παραλείπει καλλίστην τῆς τέχνης θεωρίαν; ἐχρῆν οὖν αὐτὸν μηδὲ περὶ τοῦ σπληνὸς εἰρηκέναι τι, μηδ᾽ ἀσχημονεῖν ὑπὸ τῆς τεχνικῆς φύσεως ὄργανον τηλικοῦτον μάτην ἡγούμενον κατεσκευάσθαι. καὶ μὴν οὐχ Ἱπποκράτης μόνον ἢ Πλάτων, οὐδέν τι χείρους Ἐρασιστράτου περὶ φύσιν ἄνδρες, ἕν τι τῶν ἐκκαθαιρόντων τὸ αἷμα καὶ τοῦτ᾽ εἶναί φασι τὸ σπλάγχνον, ἀλλὰ καὶ μυρίοι σὺν αὐτοῖς ἄλλοι τῶν παλαιῶν ἰατρῶν τε καὶ φιλοσόφων. *Nat. Fac.* II.9 (II 132,3–15 K), adapted from a translation by Brock.

37 See chapter 2, section 1.

38 ... ὑπὸ τὸν μαζὸν καὶ ἐς τὸν σπλῆνα καὶ ἐς τὸν νεφρόν, ... καὶ ἐκ τῶν πλευρέων ἄνωθεν ἡ μὲν ἐς τὸν σπλῆνα ἀφικνεῖται. ἡ δὲ ἐς τὸ ἧπαρ, ... *Nat. Hom.* 11, CMG I 1,3, pp. 194,13 and 196,3–4 Jouanna (VI 58,18 and 60,7–8 L), translation by Jones.

able to receive blood and other fluids as they pass through the vessels. However, there is no mention of the function of the spleen to cleanse the blood of waste material, let alone a specific mechanism to attract and remove black bile. But even this minor reference to the spleen in this treatise is in jeopardy, as we find that Galen regarded this part of *On the Nature of Man* as inauthentic.[39] Therefore, if we are directed towards this treatise then such a reference in *On the Natural Faculties* could be misleading, as there is no such material relating to the function of the spleen.

However, Galen does also refer to other, unnamed, Hippocratic treatises to support his statement relating to Hippocrates' opinion on the function of the spleen. It is possible in the passage from *On the Natural Faculties* quoted earlier (see pages 114–115 above), that Galen might be suggesting that the content relating to the humours in *On the Nature of Man* should be read in conjunction with material on the spleen in other Hippocratic texts in order to obtain a better understanding of Hippocrates' view of the function of this organ to cleanse the blood of black bile. We can find several other references to the anatomical position of the spleen in relation to other organs and the connecting blood vessels in the Hippocratic Corpus. For example, two passages in *On Diseases I* provide some information about the location of the spleen and the associated splenic vessel.[40] But, it is likely that Galen does not consider *On Diseases I* to be a genuine Hippocratic treatise, and we do not find any reference by Galen to this passage.[41] There is a large amount of material on the position and blood vessel connections of the spleen in both *On Places in Man* and *On the Nature of Bones*.[42] However, in his *Commentary on Epidemics II*, Galen discusses the anatomical information on the spleen in *On Places in Man* and *On the Nature of Bones* and associates them with the material on the spleen found in *On the Nature of Man*.[43] When it comes to *On the Nature of Bones*, we find that Galen

---

39   *PHP*, VI.3.27–31 CMG V 4,1,2 pp. 378,36–380,24 De Lacy (V 527,17–529,13 K); *HNH*, II.6, CMG V 9,1, pp. 71,4–7; 72,10–16 Mewaldt (XV 138,5–9 and 140,11–18 K). See also *Hipp. Epid. II*, CMG V 10,1 p. 311,15–22 Pfaff (from the Arabic): "We find that the information about the anatomy of the veins, which is in the book *On the Nature of Man* (11, CMG I 1,3, pp. 192,15–196,15 Jouanna (VI 58,1–60,19 L)) [is] not correct." (*Finden wir ja doch, dass die Angaben über die Anatomie der Venen, welche er in der Schrift Über die Natur des Menschen ... nicht richtig sind.*) See Anastassiou and Irmer, 1997, volume II.1, p. 368. See also chapter 2, section 3 above.

40   *Morb. I*, XXVI and XXVIII (VI 194,6–12 and 196,9–22 L).

41   See chapter 2, section 3 above.

42   *Loc. Hom.* III (VI 282,16–25 L); *Oss.* II; VIII; IX–X and XVIII (IX 168,17–170,2; 174,4–12; IX 174,13–180,23 L; 192,17–194,20 L).

43   *Hipp. Epid. II*, CMG V 10,1 p. 311,15–22 Pfaff (see footnote 39 above). See Anastassiou and Irmer, 1997, volume II.1, p. 368. Galen doubted the authenticity of *On Places in Man* any-

considered the majority of this treatise as authentic. This is in contrast to *On Places in Man*, which he considered to be inauthentic. However, from my analysis earlier, it is possible that Galen may be quoting from this text and associating some parts of it with the work of Hippocrates.[44]

Therefore, we can see that, in general, Galen was not impressed by some of these early attempts at presenting the anatomy of the body, including the location of the spleen and its connections to other organs by certain blood vessels. We have seen that Galen had explained all of what he considered to be the correct anatomical and physiological information about the spleen in detail in his *On the Utility of the Parts* (see page 107 above). Further to this, analysis of *On the Nature of Man* and other treatises from the extant Hippocratic Corpus shows that there is no justification for Galen's statements that both Asclepiades and Erasistratus could have obtained information on Hippocrates' theory of the function of the spleen to cleanse the blood of black bile. This means that Galen is manipulating the actual content of Hippocratic texts when he attacks both Asclepiades and Erasistratus on their inability to follow Hippocrates' views about the relationship between black bile and the spleen.

In his challenge to Erasistratus on the correct theory regarding the function of the spleen and black bile for the health of the body, Galen also names Plato as an authoritative source for this topic. We know that Plato regarded the spleen as an organ that purifies the blood, as in the *Timaeus* the spleen is said to cleanse (καθαίρουσα) the impurities (ἀκαθαρσίαι) that are produced in the body during illness (νόσους) (see page 111 above). We find that Plato does not specifically mention the black bile humour, and so his theory of the function of the spleen applies to a wider range of harmful substances in the blood. Galen does not draw attention to the absence of a specific reference to the spleen's cleansing of black bile in Plato's writing. However, in *On the Doctrines of Hippocrates and Plato* Galen is not constructing an argument in defence of black bile and the role of the spleen specifically to attract this humour. This is in contrast to *On the Natural Faculties* and *On Black Bile* where he does want to emphasise the function of the spleen in relation to black bile. Galen's strategy in these treatises is to inform his readers that Plato is in agreement with Galen's view that the spleen has a function of attracting black bile. In the passage from *On the Natural Faculties* quoted earlier (see pages 114–115 above), Galen extends the author-

---

way, but he did consider *On the Nature of Bones* to be a genuine work by Hippocrates. However, like parts of *On the Nature of Man*, Galen would not believe that Hippocrates wrote this passage about the blood vessels and the spleen in *On the Nature of Bones*.

44   See chapter 2, sections 3 above and pages 121–122 below.

ities on the relationship between the spleen and black bile to other physicians and doctors. This may include physicians such as Diocles and Rufus of Ephesus, but unfortunately we do not have any passages that come directly from their works that have information about the function of the spleen to remove black bile.[45]

There is another interesting remark that Galen makes in this passage from *On the Natural Faculties*. We find that when Galen chastises Erasistratus for not following Hippocrates' views of the spleen, he says that Erasistratus has 'stultified himself by holding that an artistic Nature would have prepared so large an organ for no purpose' (ἀσχημονεῖν ὑπὸ τῆς τεχνικῆς φύσεως ὄργανον τηλικοῦτον μάτην ἡγούμενον κατεσκευάσθαι). We can find a similar statement in another part of this text:

> At this point, also, I would gladly have been able to ask Erasistratus whether his "artistic" Nature has not constructed any organ for clearing away a humour [black bile] such as this. For whilst there are two organs for the excretion of urine, and another of considerable size for that of yellow bile, does the humour which is more pernicious than these wander about persistently in the veins mingled with the blood?[46]

Galen's concept of why the body and the different organs function in a certain way is part of his overall comprehensive teleological theory of the universe and all the things within it.[47] Here Galen is pointing out that Nature has constructed the spleen for a purpose, which is to cleanse the body of non-ideal natural black bile. This is comparable to *On Black Bile*, where we are told that the theory of

---

45   We find that van der Eijk includes this passage from *On the Natural Faculties* as part of fragment 27 that refers to the work of Diocles of Carystus. F27[11] (van der Eijk) = Gal. *Nat. Fac.* II.9 (II 132,12–134,16 K). There are a few fragments that refer to the spleen in what we have on the work of Rufus of Ephesus, but these are only about the issues with disease of the spleen and how to treat it and not about its function in removing black bile from the blood: F21[9] (Pormann) = ar Rāzī, *Comprehensive Book*; F66[14] and [20] = Ibn Sarābiyūn ibn Ibrāhīm, *Important Chapters on the Medicine of the Masters*, ch. 9, Rufus, *Case Notes* 1.

46   Ηὐξάμην οὖν κἀνταῦθ' ἐρωτῆσαι δύνασθαι τὸν Ἐρασίστρατον, εἰ μηδὲν ὄργανον ἡ τεχνικὴ φύσις ἐδημιούργησε καθαρτικὸν τοῦ τοιούτου χυμοῦ, ἀλλὰ τῶν μὲν οὔρων ἄρα τῆς διακρίσεώς ἐστιν ὄργανα δύο καὶ τῆς ξανθῆς χολῆς ἕτερον οὐ σμικρόν, ὁ δὲ τούτων κακοηθέστερος χυμὸς ἁλᾶται διὰ παντὸς ἐν ταῖς φλεψὶν ἀναμεμιγμένος τῷ αἵματι. *Nat. Fac.* II.9 (II 131,11–17 K), translation by Brock.

47   For example, Galen provides the reason for the structure of all the organs in the human body from a teleological perspective throughout his *On the Utility of the Parts*. See chapter 2, section 1 above.

purgation of the humours that we find in *On the Nature of Man* proves that the body must be designed to have an organ to manage non-ideal natural black bile in the body, which Galen identifies as the spleen.[48] In this way, Galen is using both the appeal to teleology and a comparison between the potentially dangerous non-ideal natural black bile with other substances, such as yellow bile and urine. This combines information from a theoretical position with that of observational evidence. Therefore, Galen has a logical argument, supported by empirical evidence, to refute Erasistratus' position regarding the useful function of the spleen in the body. However, Galen is not always consistent with this concept, as he criticised Erasistratus' denial of a teleological explanation for the presence of bile in the body, but ignored a similar argument by Aristotle on the status of bile.[49] We have a similar situation for the spleen, as Galen again has left out any reference to Aristotle's *Parts of Animals*, where the status of the spleen is discussed in relation to that of the liver:

> The spleen owes its existence to the liver being placed somewhat over to the right-hand side of the body: this makes the spleen a necessity in a way, though not an urgent one, for all animals.[50]

Aristotle's explanation is that the spleen is only a 'necessity' for some animals and even in the case with the highest forms of life such as human beings; the spleen's function is related to that of the liver for the concoction of food, where the liver is the dominant part of this combined organ and the presence of the spleen is explained more on the basis of its anatomical symmetry than by its actual function.[51] However, Galen's claim is that Erasistratus acknowledges the existence of such parts of the body as bile and the spleen, but does not assign a function or use to them. Galen is drawing upon his more comprehensive teleology, according to which almost all parts of the body must have an end-directed purpose.[52] But why does Galen focus on Erasistratus' view of bile and the spleen and ignore similar material in Aristotle's writing? Galen's stance here is related

---

48   *At. Bil.* 7, CMG V 4,1,1, p. 87,3–15 De Boer (V 135,4–136,1 K).

49   *Nat. Fac.* II.2 (II 78,10–16 K); Aristotle, *PA*, IV.2, 677a12–17. See von Staden, 1997b: 185 and 193; Vegetti, 1999: 386; Hankinson, 2008b: 227.

50   Διὰ δὲ τὸ τὴν θέσιν ἔχειν τὸ ἧπαρ ἐν τοῖς δεξιοῖς μᾶλλον ἡ τοῦ σπληνὸς γέγονε φύσις, ὥστ' ἀναγκαῖον μέν πως, μὴ λίαν δ' εἶναι πᾶσι τοῖς ζῴοις. Aristotle, *PA*, III.7, 670a1–3, translation by Forster.

51   Aristotle, *PA*, III.7, 669b13–670b23 and III.4, 666a26–28. See Hankinson, 1994a: 1757–1774; von Staden, 1997b: 193–197.

52   *UP*, V.3; V.16; XI.14 (III 346,4–16; 406,11–15 and 908,13–909,13 K).

firstly to his polemic in *On the Natural Faculties*, where he is arguing against Erasistratus and the Erasistrateans and so they will be the focus for the evidence
that he uses against them. In this argument Galen will not want to criticise Aristotle in the same context as his criticism of Erasistratus because Galen wants
to keep Aristotle as an authority to support his work and does not want to associate him with the Erasistrateans.[53]

But, there is also the case that Aristotle had given the spleen a secondary
cause in the body. This is similar to Galen's concept of the role of the jejunum,
which he says does not have an actual 'use' (χρεία) for the organism, but it follows by necessity on parts which do have a purpose.[54] However, Galen would
not agree with Aristotle on a secondary role for the spleen, as he regards this
organ as being specifically designed for its purpose of managing non-ideal natural black bile in the body. However, this identification of a secondary purpose
for the spleen would not be completely incompatible with Galen's teleological framework and could be part of what he considers as the incomplete or
inferior explanation by Aristotle, which we find in Galen's remarks in *On the
Utility of the Parts*. So, Galen did not consider Aristotle's teleology within the
sphere of biology as complete, as in this treatise, he tells us that he is writing
a more complete version of the 'usefulness' of all the parts of the body, which
Aristotle was unable to do.[55] But it would not benefit Galen's argument to raise
the issue that Aristotle had also rejected the purpose of the spleen. In fact, this
might harm his argument, as in treatises such as *On the Natural Faculties*, Galen
uses Aristotle to support his arguments against Erasistratus and Asclepiades, as
he wants to include Aristotle as one of the authorities for his presentation of
a biological theory, which is based on the qualities, elements and humours.[56]
Another related issue with Galen's presentation of his teleological argument
for the explanation of the design of all the organs and important substances in
the body, is that he regards Hippocrates as being in agreement with this comprehensive teleological view. However, we find that Galen cannot point to any
of the Hippocratic treatises to support this assertion about Hippocrates' teleology.[57] Therefore, this is another example of Galen manipulating the treatises
in the Hippocratic writings, and other authorities such as Aristotle, to make it

---

53   Von Staden, 1997b: 204–206.
54   *UP*, V.3; V.16; XI.14 (III 346,4–16; 406,11–15 and 908,13–909,13 K). See Schiefsky, 2007: 392
      (note 48).
55   *UP*, I.8; VIII.3 (III 16,7–21,16; 620,4–621,8 K). See May, 1968: 10; Hankinson, 1992: 3510; Flem-
      ming, 2009: 76–77; Gill, 2010: 31–33; van der Eijk, 2012: 266.
56   For example, *Nat. Fac.* I.2; I.3 (II 4,13–5,11; 7,15–9,6 K).
57   See chapter 2, section 1 above.

appear that there is a clear development of a biological theory of the body. This includes the purposeful design of the spleen to attract non-ideal natural black bile, which begins with the work of Hippocrates and is continued by certain physicians and philosophers and is then fully developed by Galen himself.

4 Diseases of the Spleen in Relation to the Harmful Nature of Black Bile

We have seen that Galen regarded the spleen as a very important organ for the maintenance of our health. Therefore, in his biological theory, any damage to the spleen would cause serious harm to the body. This is shown from a passage relating to the problem of the spleen becoming diseased in *On the Natural Faculties*:

> Now, all of these the high and mighty Erasistratus affected to despise, and he neither contradicted them nor even so much as mentioned their opinion. Hippocrates, indeed, says that the spleen wastes in those where the body swells to a large size, and all those physicians also who base themselves on experience agree with this. Again, in those cases in which the spleen is large and is increasing from internal suppuration, it destroys the body and fills it with evil humours; this again is agreed on, not only by Hippocrates, but also by Plato and many others, including the Empiric physicians.[58]

We can see that Galen names Plato here as an authority on information relating to the harm that may be caused to the spleen. In fact, we can find a reference to this issue in Plato's *Timaeus*, where we are informed that the spleen can 'grow large and festered' (μέγας καὶ ὕπουλος αὐξάνεται), which is found in the passage I quoted earlier (see page 111 above). But the focus of this passage is on Galen's observation that Hippocrates has described cases where the spleen 'wastes' (φθίνει) and the body 'swells' (θάλλει), indicating a close connection between the spleen and the body as a whole. When the body is seen to swell up during

---

58 ὧν ἁπάντων προσποιησάμενος ὑπερφρονεῖν ὁ γενναῖος Ἐρασίστρατος οὔτ' ἀντεῖπεν οὔθ' ὅλως τῆς δόξης αὐτῶν ἐμνημόνευσε. καὶ μὴν ὅσοις γε τὸ σῶμα θάλλει, τούτοις ὁ σπλὴν φθίνει, φησὶν Ἱπποκράτης, καὶ οἱ ἀπὸ τῆς ἐμπειρίας ὁρμώμενοι πάντες ὁμολογοῦσιν ἰατροί. καὶ ὅσοις γ' αὖ μέγας καὶ ὕπουλος αὐξάνεται, τούτοις καταφθείρει τε καὶ κακόχυμα τὰ σώματα τίθησιν, ὡς καὶ τοῦτο πάλιν οὐχ Ἱπποκράτης μόνον ἀλλὰ καὶ Πλάτων ἄλλοι τε πολλοὶ καὶ οἱ ἀπὸ τῆς ἐμπειρίας ὁμολογοῦσιν ἰατροί. *Nat. Fac.* II.9 (II 132,4–133,6 K), adapted from a translation by Brock.

an illness, then the spleen is thought to be in a bad state and is wasting away. If we search the Hippocratic Corpus, we can find a similar passage in *On Places in Man*:

> Water entering the omentum: When the spleen is enlarged as the result of fever—this happens simultaneously with the body becoming lean, since the same process makes both the spleen swell and the body waste—when the body is lean and the spleen swells and the omentum wastes along with the body, then the fat that is in the omentum melts.[59]

I believe that it is likely that Galen is referring to this section of *On Places in Man* when he tells us what Hippocrates says in the passage from *On the Natural Faculties* quoted above.[60] If this is the case, then Galen has conveniently ignored the fact that he does not believe that Hippocrates wrote this text, as he does not generally acknowledge the Hippocratic authenticity of *On Places in Man*.[61] It is possible that Galen wants to use this treatise as evidence from the authority of Hippocrates in his argument against the Erasistrateans. This passage from *On Places in Man* is also important to support his claim that there is agreement between Hippocrates and Plato on the way that the spleen wastes during illness.

Galen does use other Hippocratic treatises when he discusses cases of illness from an enlarged spleen. For example, in *On the Doctrines of Hippocrates and Plato*, he cites one of the passages from the *Aphorisms* and tells us he will use Hippocrates' exact words and the quote he uses contains information that

---

59   Ὕδωρ ἐς τὸ ἐπίπλοον· ἐπὴν ὁ σπλὴν ὑπὸ πυρετοῦ μέγας γένηται, γίνεται δὲ ὅταν τὸ σῶμα λεπτυνθῇ, τοῖσι γὰρ αὐτοῖσιν ὅ τε σπλὴν θάλλει καὶ τὸ σῶμα φθίνει· ὅταν δὲ τὸ σῶμα λεπτὸν ᾖ καὶ ὁ σπλὴν θάλλῃ καὶ τὸ ἐπίπλοον ἅμα τῷ σώματι λεπτυνθῇ, ἡ πιμελὴ ἡ ἐν τῷ ἐπιπλόῳ ἐστί, τήκεται· *Loc. Hom.* XXIV, (VI 314,19–316,10 L), adapted from a translation by Potter.

60   This is based on analysis by Anastassiou and Irmer, which shows that this is the only place in the extant Hippocratic Corpus where θάλλει and φθίνει are used to describe the spleen and the body. However, it is not clear why the two verbs, 'swell' (θάλλει) and 'waste' (φθίνει), are swapped relative to the body and spleen in *On the Natural Faculties* compared with *On Places in Man*. This could be intentional by Galen himself, or perhaps due to a copyist error in either of these treatises. However, as we do not find this type of association in any other extant text within the Hippocratic Corpus, it is the most likely reference for Galen's statement about Hippocrates in *On the Natural Faculties*. Further to this, we find a number of other quotes and references to *On Places in Man*, which Galen attributes to Hippocrates. For example, *Symp. Caus.* (VII 115,13–17; 176,3–13 K); *Inaeq. Int.* (VII 739,5–12 K). See Anastassiou and Irmer, 1997, II.2, pp. 249–251.

61   See chapter 2, section 3 above.

enlarged spleens are more common in the autumn.[62] However, Galen does not provide any analysis or comment about the presence of 'enlarged spleen' in this list of autumnal diseases, but this does provide an indirect connection between the spleen and black bile, as in *On the Nature of Man* the black bile humour is said to be more abundant in the autumn because it shares the qualities of cold and dry with this season.[63] We find generally that the Hippocratic physicians take note of the state of the spleen in many cases, using different terms that essentially say the same thing, which is that this organ has increased in size above the normal. For example, in *On Regimen in Acute Diseases*, the spleen is said to become grown (αὐξητικός).[64] In *Epidemics III* there is a reference to a patient's spleen being enlarged (σπλὴν ἐπήρθη).[65] Alternatively, we find in *Epidemics II* that the spleen is described simply as being large (μέγας).[66] However, Galen tends not to reference or quote many of the different observations and case studies in the Hippocratic writings on disease and abnormal growth of the spleen. In one particular case, in *On Affections*, the Hippocratic author goes into great detail about the problems that arise when a patient has a large spleen. The cause of disease is identified by either fever, or by incorrect therapy, and both phlegm and bile can become deposited in the spleen itself.[67] All of these texts are considered by Galen to be Hippocratic, but he remains silent about this material in relation to his own advice about treating disorders of the spleen. But it is certainly not the case that Galen completely ignores the Hippocratic Corpus with respect to the spleen. The enlargement of the spleen seems to be a symptom of some illnesses in which Galen identifies difficulties in the respiratory system and he quotes and makes reference to four different case studies in *Epidemics I*, *IV* and *VI*, but again he does not focus on any specific details about the function of the spleen and its purification of non-ideal natural black bile from the blood.[68]

---

62   Hippocratic Corpus, *Aph.* III.22, (IV 496,4–8 L); Gal. *PHP*, VIII.6.16–36, CMG V 4,1,2 pp. 516, 7–520,1 De Lacy (V 692,12–697,2 K); *Hipp. Aph.* III.5 (XVIIb 570,7–571,6 K). See Anastassiou and Irmer, 1997, volume II.1, p. 103 and II.2 p. 86.

63   See chapter 3, section 1 above.

64   *Acut.* LXII (17 L), (II 358,15–360,4 L).

65   *Epid. III*, case III (fourth day), (III 40,10 L). There are many other terms used such as ὑπόσπληνος (*Epid. II*, II.6, (V 86,10–11 L)), ἐπισπλήνωι (*Epid. IV*, I.35, (V 178,13–16 L)), ἔπαρσις (*Epid. VI*, II.5, (V 278,12–14 L)), σπληνώδς (*Epid. VII*, I.105, (V 456,1–5 L)), or ὀγκηρός (*Liqu.* VI (VI 130,3–11 L)).

66   *Epid. II*, II.7; 22 (V 86,16; 94,1–2 L).

67   *Aff.* XX (VI 228,20–230,22 L).

68   Hippocratic Corpus, *Epid. I*, case 1 (end); case III (fifth day, eighth day and end), (II 684,8–9; 688,13–14; 690,1–2; 690,6 L); *Epid. IV*, I.25; 27, (V 164,15–166,3; V 172,1–5 L); *Epid. VI*, III.2

We can find information on the spleen in the Hippocratic *On Humours*, another one of the treatises that Galen regarded as authentic. In this work there are some references to more general cases of the spleen, such as the case where this organ can become diseased from drinking water or in summer from an excess of bile.[69] However, this material does not identify black bile as being the problem, which is not surprising as this treatise does not contain any material on this humour.[70] Galen does not provide any comment on this particular passage, but we can see from this that the spleen was considered an important organ in the Hippocratic Corpus. Another passage, this time from *On Internal Affections*, provides more detail about the conditions that bring on a disease in the spleen:

> The first disease of the spleen: it is produced by the heat of the sun, when bile is set in motion and the spleen draws bile to itself ... Another disease of the spleen: it is produced mostly in the season of the summer; the disease is produced by blood, when the spleen becomes filled with blood, it breaks out into the cavity of the body ... Another disease of the spleen: the disease mostly occurs suddenly in spring; when the spleen takes up phlegm into itself, it immediately becomes large and hard; then it is restored to its normal state ... Another disease of the spleen: it is produced by black bile mostly in late autumn; it is produced from eating many raw vegetables and from drinking water.[71]

This is an example of all the four humours that are defined in the Hippocratic *On the Nature of Man* being used together to explain the different diseases of the spleen.[72] It appears that Galen acknowledged the Hippocratic authenticity of *On Internal Affections*, but believed it to be by a later Hippocratean rather

---

(V 292,14–294,2 L); Gal. *Diff. Resp.*, 11.10–11; 111.12–13 (VII 871,4–880,13; 951,4–959,17 K). See Anastassiou and Irmer, 1997, volume II.2, pp. 145–146, 201 and 211.

69   In *Hum.* (XII; XIII (V 492,7–16; 494,3–6 L)) both σπληνώδς and ὑπόσπληνος are used for 'disease of the spleen'.

70   See chapter 2, section 3 above.

71   Σπληνὸς ἡ πρώτη· γίνεται δὲ διὰ θερμασίην τοῦ ἡλίου, χολῆς κινηθείσης, ὅταν ἑλκύσῃ ὁ σπλὴν ἐφ' ἑωυτὸν χολήν ... Ἄλλη σπληνός· γίνεται μὲν τοῦ ἔτεος θέρεος ὥρῃ μάλιστα· ἡ δὲ νοῦσος γίνεται ἀπὸ αἵματος, ὅταν ὁ σπλὴν ἐμπλησθῇ αἵματος, ἐκρήγνυται ἐς τὴν κοιλίην ... Ἄλλη σπληνός· προσπίπτει ἡ νοῦσος μάλιστα ἦρος· ὅταν φλέγμα ἀναλάβῃ ὁ σπλὴν ἐς ἑωυτόν, μέγας παραχρῆμα γίνεται καὶ σκληρός· εἶτα αὖτις καθίσταται· ... Ἄλλη σπληνός· γίνεται μὲν μετοπώρου μάλιστα ἀπὸ χολῆς μελαίνης· γίνεται δὲ ἀπὸ λαχανοφαγίης τρωξίμων πολλῶν καὶ ἀπὸ ὑδροποσίης. *Int.* XXX; XXXII; XXXIII; XXXIV (VII 244,6–8; 248,14–16, 250,15–18; 252,6–8 L), adapted from a translation by Potter.

72   *Nat. Hom.* 4, CMG I 1,3, p. 174,2–3 Jouanna (VI 40,4–6 L).

than by Hippocrates himself.[73] However, these passages from *On Internal Affections* are not in agreement with Galen's view that the spleen only targets 'black bile' to be drawn out of the blood, as the other humours are described as being drawn to the spleen under the different environmental conditions of the seasons. But, this passage from *On Internal Affections* is consistent with the more general view that we find in Plato's writing on the spleen. Here we find that the spleen purifies the blood of general unwanted waste material, rather than specifically attracting black bile. This also shows that Galen would have some difficulty in drawing together all the information from the treatises of the Hippocratic writings, which he identifies as being Hippocratic, to show that Hippocrates had a particular theory regarding the function of the spleen and which substances it draws in to purify the blood. Instead, Galen is very selective with his sources and only provides quotations when he wants to draw the reader to a particular point he wants to make.

However, there is another example where Galen refers to a Hippocratic text to discuss the issues concerned with the diseases that can affect the spleen. Again, it is found in *On the Natural Faculties*, but this time Galen actually quotes his Hippocratic source:

> Indeed, somewhere Hippocrates says, "Dysentery, if it starts from black bile, is fatal", while that proceeding from yellow bile is not completely deadly, but most people recover from it. This proves how much more pernicious and acrid in its potentialities is black bile than yellow bile.[74]

The quote in the passage above, which Galen tells us comes from somewhere in Hippocrates' works, is actually from the Hippocratic *Aphorisms* (IV.24). It is a single line statement about the fatal impact of dysentery by black bile.[75] Just before this passage, Galen emphasises that it is clear that Erasistratus was wrong in his view that the spleen has no function because Nature would have created an organ to remove surplus black bile from the body. Therefore, this is a connection between the function of the spleen and the avoidance of dysentery that is caused by the presence of too much black bile. We can see here that Galen uses the term 'black bile' (μέλαινα χολή), rather than 'melancholic

---

73　See chapter 2, section 3 above.

74　καίτοι "Δυσεντερίη," φησί που Ἱπποκράτης, "ἢν ἀπὸ χολῆς μελαίνης ἄρξηται, θανάσιμον," οὐ μὴν ἥ γ' ἀπὸ τῆς ξανθῆς χολῆς ἀρχομένη πάντως ὀλέθριος, ἀλλ' οἱ πλείους ἐξ αὐτῆς διασῴζονται. τοσούτῳ κακοηθεστέρα τε καὶ δριμυτέρα τὴν δύναμιν ἡ μέλαινα χολὴ τῆς ξανθῆς ἐστιν. *Nat. Fac.* II.9 (II 131,17–132,3 K), adapted from a translation by Brock.

75　*Aph.* IV.24, (IV 510,9–10 L). See Anastassiou and Irmer, 1997, volume II.2, pp. 90.

humour' (μελαγχολικὸς χυμός), as μέλαινα χολή is used in the original Hippocratic source. However, the type of black bile appears to be the altered black
bile, as it is described as having dangerous and acidic properties. Galen could
also have used μελαγχολικὸς χυμός to refer to the altered black bile, as he does in
other texts such as *On Black Bile*, but it is more important for Galen to use the
same terms as the sources that he is referring to, as this will reduce any confu-
sion and allow him to align the ideas contained in these Hippocratic texts with
his own work and with other non-Hippocratic sources.

Galen also quotes this aphorism in *On Black Bile* and *On the Utility of the
Parts*, which I will be discussing later.[76] But at this point, I want to bring the
discussion back to the spleen, which in Galenic texts such as *On the Natural Faculties* and *On Black Bile*, is the organ that regulates non-ideal natural black bile
in the body. In the Hippocratic Corpus there is a strong association between
the spleen and the suffering of diseases related to dysentery. For example in
another passage from the Hippocratic *Aphorisms*:

> When persons with enlarged spleens are attacked by dysentery, if the
> dysentery that supervenes is prolonged, dropsy or lientery supervenes
> with fatal results.[77]

This is *Aph.* (VI.43), and describes a type of dysentery. Therefore, this is important for the diagnosis and prognosis of these diseases based on the condition
of the spleen. However, there is another aphorism (*Aph.* VI.48), which tells us
the following:

> In cases of enlarged spleen, dysentery supervening is a good thing.[78]

So here we have the same type of reference to an enlarged spleen, but this time
dysentery is beneficial for the patient. The difference between the two aphorisms is that in *Aph.* (VI.43) the dysentery is prolonged, which gives time for
other diseases, such as dropsy and lientery, to occur. However, in *Aph.* (VI.48)
dysentery has occurred and has flushed out harmful substances in order to alle-
viate the condition, and this is beneficial as long as the dysentery does not occur

---

76   See chapter 7, section 3 below.
77   Ὁκόσοι σπληνώδεες ὑπὸ δυσεντερίης ἁλίσκονται, τούτοισιν, ἐπιγενομένης μακρῆς τῆς δυσεντε-
      ρίης, ὕδρωψ ἐπιγίνεται ἢ λειεντερίη, καὶ ἀπόλλυνται. *Aph.* VI.43, (IV 574,2–4 L), translation by
      Jones.
78   Τοῖσι σπληνώδεσι δυσεντερίη ἐπιγενομένη, ἀγαθόν. *Aph.* VI.48, (IV 576,1 L), translation by
      Jones.

for a long time. However, Galen believes that there is a contradiction between these two aphorisms. He argues that *Aph.* (VI.48) is merely an oversight in this text and that Hippocrates himself prefers *Aph.* (VI.43), which asserts that the combination of prolonged dysentery with an enlarged spleen is an indication of a terminal case. He tells us that we should forget about *Aph.* (VI.48), as there is no need for it to be acknowledged as part of what should be remembered for medical practice.[79] Here Galen is criticising what he sees as an inconsistency between two aphorisms that are in fact telling us two different things. But, Galen wants to reinforce the notion that Hippocrates also postulated that a severe illness occurs if altered black bile is present in the body and at the same time the spleen is either damaged or unable to function properly. We have seen that if the spleen cannot remove the non-ideal natural black bile from the blood there is the potential for it to transform into altered black bile. For Galen, *Aph.* (VI.48) seems to challenge this idea and so he rejects it in favour of *Aph.* (VI.43). Therefore, Galen is selective of passages from the Hippocratic *Aphorisms*, as he wants to show that Hippocrates is in complete agreement with his own biological theory and its teleological framework.

5 Summary

The analysis of Galen's writing on the origin and management of black bile in the body emphasises the importance of understanding the way he differentiates between three different types: ideal natural, non-ideal natural and altered black bile. For example, in the case of the origin of black bile, Galen's view is that ideal natural black bile is produced from certain types of foodstuff in the blood vessels. Understanding of the distinction between the three types of black bile on the basis of their production in the body is hindered by Galen's often 'looseness of language'. Galen uses 'melancholic humour' (μελαγχολικός χυμός) and 'black bile' (μέλαινα χολή) interchangeably in *On the Natural Faculties* and *On the Utility of the Parts* when he names the type of black bile that is drawn into the spleen. This is because he cannot be so precise with his terminology of black bile in these treatises as there are situations when he needs to use μέλαινα χολή in his polemical arguments against his rivals, such as Erasistratus and Asclepiades, or in cases where he is quoting a source, such as a

---

79 For Galen's argument regarding Hippocrates' preference for Aphorism VI.43, see *Hipp. Aph.* VI.43 (XVIIIa 67,1–4 K). For Galen's rejection of Aphorism VI.48, see *Hipp. Aph.* VI.48 (XVIIIa 81,15–82,4 K). See also Anastassiou and Irmer, 1997, volume II.1, pp. 137–138.

Hippocratic text, which itself uses the term μέλαινα χολή such as the Hippocratic *Aphorisms*. Galen's strategy is to use language in the best way for his
specific argument in a particular treatise, without having a systematic framework of nomenclature that could hinder his use of different sources for his
refutation of the theories of his rivals. We can also see possible evidence of
Galen's manipulation of his sources when he wants to show that Hippocrates
is in agreement with the notion that the presence of altered black bile in the
body can be fatal. In this way, Galen is selecting material from a work that he
generally considers to be genuinely by Hippocrates, but rejecting certain passages with which he does not agree.

CHAPTER 7

The Diseases Caused by Black Bile

Now we move on to the important area of Galen's explanation of black bile as the cause of disease. At the beginning of this chapter, I will focus on Galen's writing about two specific types of disease relating to black bile. The first is the melancholy illness that by its very name has been associated with black bile in early medical theories. The second disease that I am going to write about is quartan fever. This illness is important, as it provides to be a useful insight into the way that Galen attempts to demonstrate that Hippocrates was the first to associate this fever with black bile. I will then discuss the important issues concerning some more general aspects of black bile in Galen's aetiology of disease with reference to its potential to cause terminal illness in the body.

1   Melancholy, the Black Bile Disease

The illness known as 'melancholy' is a mental disorder causing conditions such as madness and despondency.[1] The earliest references to an illness called

---

1   For example, the concept of a 'melancholic' (μελαγχολική) constitution was important in the work of the Aristotelians for the way that emotions and behaviour are produced by the physiology of the body. We find from Aristotle's writing that people with melancholic temperaments are prone to hallucinations. He refers also to black bile as a type of moisture (ὑγρός), which can affect the sight of melancholic people. This black bile, being a cold substance, affects the heart and the area surrounding it, which is also the nutritive region in Aristotle's physiological theory. For Aristotle on melancholic conditions and hallucinations, see *Div. Somn.* II, 463b17–18 and 464a33–464b1; *Mem.* 453a19–21. For Aristotle on the effect of a moisture (black bile) on people with a melancholic condition, see *HA*, III.2, 511b10–11; *Somn. Vig.* III, 457a32–34. See also van der Eijk, 2005: 141–143. Those who are considered to have melancholic constitutions are said to be more disposed than other people towards contracting melancholic types of disease. But there is a positive side to being melancholic, as extraordinary men, in such areas as philosophy, poetry and politics, tend to have melancholic temperaments. Pseudo-Aristotle, *Pr.* XXX.1, 953a10–20. Cicero wrote in his *Tusculum Dispensations* that it was an Aristotelian idea that genius is firmly connected with melancholy (*Aristoteles quidem ait omnes ingeniosos melancholicos esse*). Cicero, *Tusc.* I.80. See Flashar, 1966: 67–68. Schütrumpf points out that although there is the positive side of the effects of black bile to produce 'extraordinary men' (*Pr.* XXX.1, 953a12), this is countered by an associated tendency to suffer from illnesses caused by black bile. See Schütrumpf, 2015: 361. For a more general overview of how ancient physicians and philosophers perceived mental illness and madness, which includes conditions such as epilepsy and melancholy, see Siegel, 1968:

---

melancholia can be found in the Hippocratic Corpus, but there is no explicit
concept of a physiological theory of this disease at this stage. There is not even
a clear association with a humour, such as black bile. However, we can find
a more established theory of melancholy with a physiological basis relating
to black bile in Aristotelian sources[2] of the fourth century BCE and then later
in the writings of Rufus of Ephesus[3] and Aretaeus of Cappadocia[4] in the first
century CE. In Galen's system melancholy has a physiological basis and is associated with the black bile humour.[5] In *On Affected Parts* Galen distinguishes
between three different types of melancholy. Firstly, there is the condition
related to the hypochondrium, which begins in the region of the stomach. Secondly, there is the condition arising from an affection of the brain. Lastly, there
is a more general case of melancholy when black bile affects the whole body.
Galen provides details of all three types, where he initially describes them sep-
arately and then discusses all three as part of a development of the melancholic
illness.[6] The first type begins in the stomach:

> If, then, the first symptoms start in the stomach and if, once they have
> become stronger, they are accompanied by melancholic affections, and if
> the patient derives relief from these by laxatives, emetics, breaking wind,
> and belching, we call this disease hypochondriac and flatulent. We will
> say that its symptoms are despondency and fear ... when a melancholic
> evaporation rises upwards to the brain, like some kind of sooty or smoky
> vapour, the melancholic symptoms affect the thinking faculty.[7]

300–304; Harris, 2013: 1–23. For a study of melancholy as a form of depression, rather than
madness, in Greek philosophy and medical texts, see Kazantzidis, 2013: 245–264.

2   For more information on the Aristotelian concept of melancholy and its association with
black bile, see van der Eijk, 2005: 140.

3   For more detail on how the concept of melancholy as a disease was developed by physicians
such as Rufus of Ephesus, see Flashar, 1966: 84–104 and Pormann, 2013: 223–244.

4   Aretaeus' theory of melancholy, in contrast to the views of Galen and Rufus, allows for a purely
psychological cause for this disease, without a mechanism relating to the balance of black bile
in the body. See Flashar, 1966: 76–79 and Bell, 2014: 42, 64, 67 and 79.

5   For an overview of Galen's development of theories and treatments for different types of mental conditions, see Nutton, 2013: 119–128 and Bell, 2014: 38.

6   F5[9] (Pormann) = Isḥāq ibn ʿImrān, *On Melancholy*. This statement is the basis for the modern view that Galen used Rufus as a source for his writing on all three types of melancholy in
On Affected Parts. See Flashar, 1966: 105 and 107; Pormann, 2008: 5–6 and Bell, 2014: 42.

7   ἐὰν μὲν οὖν ἄρξηταί γε πρῶτα τὰ κατὰ τὴν γαστέρα συμπτώματα, καὶ μείζοσιν αὐτοῖς γινομέ-
νοις ἀκολουθήσῃ τὰ μελαγχολικὰ πάθη, κουφίζηταί τε ταῖς διαχωρήσεσιν καὶ τοῖς ἐμέτοις καὶ ταῖς
κάτω φύσαις καὶ ταῖς ἐρυγαῖς ὁ ἄνθρωπος, ὑποχονδριακὸν μὲν ὀνομάσομεν οὕτως γε καὶ φυσῶδες
τὸ νόσημα, συμπτώματα δὲ εἶναι φήσομεν αὐτοῦ, τήν τε δυσθυμίαν καὶ τὸν φόβον· ... νῦν ἐπὶ τὸν

This is referred to as the hypochondriac melancholy, which can be found also in the sources attributed to Rufus of Ephesus' writing on this type of disease. It appears that this was the subject of Rufus' *On Melancholy*, where the origin of this melancholy is in the place below the rib-cartilage (the hypochondrium) and near to an opening to the stomach.[8] However, in *On Affected Parts*, Galen does not quote or refer to the work of Rufus, but instead discusses Diocles' theory on the disease known as melancholia. Galen quotes long sections from Diocles' *Affection, Cause, Treatment*, which describe the symptoms relating to the hypochondriac melancholy. Galen criticises Diocles for not including the most important symptoms for conditions that are covered under a broader definition of melancholy diseases. These symptoms relate to mental disturbances, such as fear and depression, which Galen believes Diocles did not state because they may be ascertained from the name of the disease itself.[9] When it comes to analysing what Diocles has said about the hypochondriac melancholy, Galen believes that Diocles was unable to account properly for psychological disorders associated with this illness. Diocles favoured the cardio-centric location of the ruling part of the soul, which, as van der Eijk points out, was in conflict with Galen's own view. Another point of interest is that Galen does refer to the presence of phlegm, but not to the absence of black bile, in the explanation of the cause of hypochondriac melancholy in Diocles' writing on this topic.[10] In addition to the material by Diocles, Galen also references passages from the Hippocratic writings. For example, he quotes from the Hippocratic *Aphorisms*, as evidence that these symptoms are essential for a correct diagnosis of hypochondriac melancholy.[11] However, there is another Hippocratic text, *Koan Prognoses*, which Galen identifies as containing genuine Hippocratic doctrine, that has information on patients that have become 'deranged in a melancholic manner' (τῶν ἐξισταμένων μελαγχολικῶς).[12] We find that these passages from

---

ἐγκέφαλον ἀναφερομένης τῆς μελαγχολικῆς ἀναθυμιάσεως, οἷον αἰθαλώδους τινὸς, ἢ καπνώδους ἀναθυμιάσεως, τὰ μελαγχολικὰ γενήσεται περὶ τὴν διάνοιαν συμπτώματα. *Loc. Aff.* III.10 (VIII 192,1–5; 189,7–11 K), translation by van der Eijk.

8   F5[7–9] (Pormann) = Isḥāq ibn 'Imrān, *On Melancholy*; F6[1–7] (Pormann) = Ya'qūb al-Kaskarī, *Compendium on Medicine*; F7[1–2] (Pormann) = Ibn Sīnā, *Canon of Medicine*. See Siegel, 1968: 303; Pormann, 2008: 5.

9   F109 (van der Eijk) = Gal. *Loc. Aff.* III.10 (VIII 185,14–189,2 K). However, it has been pointed out by van der Eijk that the term 'melancholy' (μελαγχολία) does not actually occur in the passages from Diocles that Galen quotes. See van der Eijk, 2001: 217; 2008: 168.

10   See van der Eijk, 2001: 216–224; 2008: 167–169.

11   Hippocratic Corpus, *Aph.* VI.23 (IV 568,11–12 L); Gal. *Loc. Aff.* III.10 (VIII 188,3–7 K). This aphorism is also quoted by Galen in *On Causes of Symptoms* (II.VII.2 (VII 202,18–203,8 K)). See Anastassiou and Irmer, 1997, volume II.2, pp. 101–102; Jouanna, 2012a: 234–235.

12   *Coac.* 87; 92; 93; 128 (V 602,11–12; 602,17–18; 602,18–20; 610,1–3 L).

Koan Prognoses do not specifically mention the black bile humour as the cause of this condition, but then the same is true for the passage from *Aphorisms*. It seems that Galen prefers to quote and reference material from *Aphorisms* in relation to similar material from another Hippocratic text such as *Koan Prognoses*. This shows that Galen relies upon one of his 'core' genuine Hippocratic texts to provide the critical material to prove his point. Galen does this even though there is no reference to hypochondriac melancholy in *Aphorisms* or in any other extant Hippocratic work, while there is a large amount of information on the hypochondriac melancholy in the material associated with Rufus of Ephesus.

The next type of melancholy is acquired if the patient experiences prolonged and intense symptoms of fear and despondency:

> Yet when the symptoms characteristic of melancholy manifest themselves to a great extent, whilst there is little or no suffering in the stomach, one must assume that the brain is primarily affected, since black bile has gathered there ... But when it [this thick melancholic humour] is present in excess in the very body of the brain, it causes melancholy, just as the other kind of humour of black bile, the one that has arisen as a result of the burning of yellow bile, results in bestial hallucinations, both without fever and with fever when it fills the brain excessively.[13]

When it comes to the effect of black bile on the brain, Galen makes a distinction between the two types of this humour. It is important for Galen to be clear about this, as the thick, non-ideal natural black bile can affect the brain without causing severe ulceration and corrosion of the organic matter. This means that it can be treated by a therapy, such as a specific type of diet. In the case of the altered black bile causing bestial hallucinations, Galen does not supply any further information, but we would assume that given the harmful nature of this type of black bile the patient would also suffer from the corrosive effects of the acidic black bile on the body, which could indicate a terminal prognosis (see section 3 below). However, earlier, when I discussed Galen's use of altered

---

13   ὅταν δὲ τὰ μὲν τῆς μελαγχολίας ἴδια συμπτώματα φαίνηται μεγάλα, κατὰ δὲ τὴν κοιλίαν ἤτοι μηδὲν, ἢ σμικρά, τὸν ἐγκέφαλον ἡγητέον ἐπὶ τούτων πρωτοπαθεῖν, ἠθροισμένης ἐν αὐτῷ μελαίνης χολῆς ... ὅτ' ἂν δ' ἐν αὐτῷ πλεονάσῃ τῷ τοῦ ἐγκεφάλου σώματι, μελαγχολίαν ἐργάζεται, καθάπερ ὁ ἕτερος χυμὸς τῆς μελαίνης χολῆς, ὁ κατωπτημένης τῆς ξανθῆς χολῆς γενόμενος, τὰς θηριώδεις παραφροσύνας ἀποτελεῖ χωρὶς πυρετοῦ τε καὶ σὺν πυρετῷ, πλεονάζων ἐν τῷ σώματι τοῦ ἐγκεφάλου. *Loc. Aff.* III.10; III.9 (VIII 192,8–11; 177,15–178,3 K), translation by van der Eijk. See also Flashar, 1966: 107.

forms of black bile which are produced by the burning of black bile, yellow bile or blood, there were some references to the heating of the humours in the writing attributed to Rufus of Ephesus.[14] The hypochondriac melancholy attributed to Rufus can be considered as two different conditions in the body: either it is caused by a natural mixture or it comes from some acquired state, such as from a bad diet. In the second case we find that a person can become at first angry then sad and afraid. This is explained by the cooking of yellow bile producing rage, which when fully burnt up, cools to create the fear and sadness. This could be a potential source for Galen's view of melancholy in *On Affected Parts*, as there are similarities between the two accounts. Both Galen and Rufus refer to the burning of yellow bile that causes different symptoms to melancholy. Galen's burnt yellow bile is a form of altered black bile and causes 'bestial hallucinations'. Rufus' theory is similar, with the cooking of yellow bile causing a person to be bolder (θρασύτερος) and quick to anger (ὀργιλώτερος) and he implies that this can occur during the melancholy illness, lasting as long as the yellow bile is burning. The subsequent cooling process allows the melancholic symptoms to return. The material we have from Aëtius that discusses Rufus' theory of melancholy does not refer to this burnt yellow bile as an altered form of black bile, but an earlier passage does say that the humours become black through excessive heat and drying out.[15] Therefore, Rufus' explanation of the harmful effects of burnt yellow bile could be a possible source for Galen on this topic. However, Galen does not directly refer to Rufus when he writes about this harmful substance produced from the burning of yellow bile in the body.

Towards the end of his discussion of melancholy in *On Affected Parts*, Galen emphasises the importance of understanding the way that the humours can cause mental illness:

> For the best doctors and philosophers are agreed that the humours and in general the mixture of the body cause alteration to the activities of the soul. I myself demonstrated this in one treatise, in which I showed *That the Faculties of the Soul Follow the Mixtures of the Body*. This is why those who do not know the power of the humours do not dare to write on melancholy, among whom are the followers of Erasistratus.[16]

---

14   See chapter 4, section 2 above.
15   F11[21–24] (Pormann) = Aëtius, *Medical Books*, vi. 9 (frg. 70 (Daremberg)).
16   ὅτι γὰρ οἵ τε χυμοὶ καὶ ὅλως ἡ τοῦ σώματος κρᾶσις ἀλλοιοῖ τὰς ἐνεργείας τῆς ψυχῆς, ὡμολόγη-
     ται τοῖς ἀρίστοις ἰατροῖς τε καὶ φιλοσόφοις, ἐμοί τε δι' ἑνὸς ὑπομνήματος ἀποδέδεικται, καθ' ὃ
     ταῖς τοῦ σώματος κράσεσιν ἀκολουθούσας ἀπέδειξα τὰς τῆς ψυχῆς δυνάμεις· ὅθεν οὐδὲ γράψαι

We see that Galen advertises his work on the way that the mixtures of the qualities (hot, cold, dry and wet) can affect the 'activities of the soul'. If we investigate *The Faculties of the Soul Follow the Mixtures of the Body*, there are three places where melancholy is discussed. Firstly, Galen confesses that he does not know the underlying mechanism that causes certain types of mental illness in the brain:

> ... nor (have I discovered) why when there is a build-up of yellow bile in the brain we are brought into a state of derangement; or when there is a build-up of black bile, into melancholy; ...[17]

One point to note is that in this passage Galen uses 'black bile' (μέλαινα χολή), rather than 'melancholic humour' (μελαγχολικὸς χυμός) for the type of black bile that causes melancholy. This is an example of Galen using 'loose' language, as he has stated in *On Affected Parts* that the non-ideal natural black bile should be properly called μελαγχολικὸς χυμός, rather than μέλαινα χολή.[18] The second reference to melancholy in *The Faculties of the Soul Follow the Mixtures of the Body* provides a description of the effects of this illness on the soul, such as it causing distress and a lack of resolve and spirit. Lastly, melancholy is given as an example, along with phrenitis and madness, of the effect of disease in the body on the soul.[19] Galen does not say very much in *On Affected Parts* about the third type of melancholy, which occurs when non-ideal natural black bile has become dominant in all parts of the body. What he does say is within the context of advice to doctors on the importance of correct diagnosis for the best treatment to be applied. Therefore, it is important to be able to know whether there is a large amount of non-ideal natural black bile in just the brain, or in the whole body. This is because in the latter, therapeutic treatments do not work, and instead phlebotomy must be used.[20] Finally, we find that in his *Commentary on On the Nature of Man*, Galen refers to a physical theory that associates each of the humours with a particular character of the soul, where a 'melancholic constitution' (μελαγχολικός), which occurs when there is a predominance of the black bile humour in the body, causes a person to be 'steady'

τι περὶ μελαγχολίας ἐτόλμησαν οἱ τὴν τῶν χυμῶν δύναμιν ἀγνοήσαντες, ἐξ ὧν εἰσι καὶ οἱ περὶ τὸν Ἐρασίστρατον. *Loc. Aff.* III.10 (VIII 191,8–14 K), translation by van der Eijk.

17 ... ὥσπερ γ' οὐδὲ διὰ τί χολῆς μὲν ξανθῆς ἐν ἐγκεφάλῳ πλεοναζούσης εἰς παραφροσύνην ἑλκόμεθα, διὰ τί δὲ τῆς μελαίνης εἰς μελαγχολίαν, ... *QAM*, III (IV 776,19–777,3 K), translation by Singer.

18 See chapter 4, section 1 above.

19 *QAM*, III; V (IV 779,13–21; 788,11–13 K).

20 *Loc. Aff.* III.10 (VIII 182,6–12; 192,11–193,1 K). See Flashar, 1966: 107.

(ἑδραῖος) and 'firm' (βέβαιος).[21] Galen does not provide any more information on this theory here or in any other of his extant treatises. This is also the only place in *Commentary on On the Nature of Man* where Galen uses μελαγχολικὸς χυμός and it could be a similar reference to the effect of the non-ideal natural black bile on the brain, as we find in *On Affected Parts*.

We find also in *On Affected Parts* that epilepsy can be associated with black bile:

> Just like the thick phlegmatic humour, this thick melancholic humour likewise sometimes causes instances of epilepsy, because it is contained in the places where the cavities of the brain, whether the middle or the posterior cavity, have their exit channels.[22]

Galen explains a little later in the text that when thick humours, like phlegm and non-ideal natural black bile, are present in large amounts in the brain, they can cause damage to it either as an 'organic' (ὀργανικός) or as a 'homogeneous' (ὁμοιομέρεια) system.[23] This means that Galen is describing the brain in two ways, which explain the cause of different types of disease. The 'organic' system is the collection of different parts of the brain, such as the various types of vessels that allow the brain to function. The thick humours affect this 'organic' system when they obstruct the blood vessels. The 'homogeneous' system describes the brain as a uniform structure of matter. It is affected when its overall qualitative mixture is altered by the presence of the thick humours. Galen supports his explanation with a quote from *Epidemics VI*, which claims that people with a melancholic condition can become epileptic and vice-versa. Transition from one illness to the other is said to be dependent on whether the illness (ἀρρώστημα) affects the body (σῶμα), which causes epilepsy, or the mind (διάνοια), which produces melancholy. Galen interprets this Hippocratic text as showing that there are cases where epilepsy can be produced by non-ideal natural black bile, as well as by the thick phlegmatic humour. But there is a difference, as epilepsy that has been caused by non-ideal natural black bile can transform into melancholy, which is not the case when it is produced by the thick phlegmatic humour. Further to this, Galen uses this passage from *Epi-*

---

21   *HNH*, I.40, CMG V 9,1, p. 51,13–16 Mewaldt (XV 97,10–13 K).

22   ὥσπερ δ' ὁ παχὺς χυμὸς τοῦ φλέγματος, οὕτω καὶ οὗτος παχὺς χυμὸς ὁ μελαγχολικὸς ἐπιλη-ψίας ποτ' ἐργάζεται κατὰ τὰς ἐκροὰς τῶν ἐν ἐγκεφάλῳ κοιλιῶν ἰσχόμενος, ἤτοι τῆς μέσης, ἢ τῆς ὄπισθεν· *Loc. Aff.* III.9 (VIII 177,12–15 K), translation by van der Eijk.

23   For more information on Galen's theory about the importance of understanding the different levels of matter in the body, see *Morb. Diff.* III.1–IV.5 (VI 841,1–848,3 K).

demics VI to show that Hippocrates also viewed the condition of the soul (ψυχή) as dependent on the mixture of the qualities. Galen believes that this confirms that there are two mechanisms for bile to affect the brain, one that can hinder the function of this organ, and the other that can alter the homoeomerous substance of the brain. However, all that the passage from *Epidemics VI* tells us is that there are two related diseases, epilepsy and melancholy, with the possibility of change from one to the other, which is based on some unspecified affection of either the body or the mind. In this passage there is no mention of any humours, phlegm, bile or black bile, and it does not even refer to the qualities.[24]

2   Quartan Fever, the Black Bile Fever

There are many different types of fever discussed in ancient medicine. Some are differentiated by the length of time between bouts of illness, such as the continuous, quotidian, tertian and quartan fevers. Out of these fevers, we find that Galen considers black bile to be the cause of quartan fevers and he is very critical of anyone who either denies this is the case, or postulates any alternative causes for this type of periodic fever. For example, in *On the Doctrines of Hippocrates and Plato*, Galen criticises Plato for presenting a theory of the cause of the different fevers based on the cosmic elements, which he felt was inferior to the cause of fevers from the individual humours that he claims was developed by Hippocrates:

> Therefore (Plato) neglected to examine these same things, and even more, the things that Hippocrates wrote about the diseases that predominate at each age and in each season. If he had paid attention to them he would not have written these words: "Now the body that has fallen sick chiefly from an excess of fire produces continuous heats and fevers; that from air, quotidian fevers; that from water, tertian fevers, because water is more sluggish than air and fire; and that from earth, in the fourth place, is the most sluggish of all; being purged in fourfold periods of time and producing quartan fevers, it barely manages to escape." (Plato's) first error in this account was to explain the causes of periodic fevers in terms of the elements common to all bodies rather than the elements of blooded animals.

---

24   Hippocratic Corpus, *Epid VI*, VIII.31 (V 354,19–356,3 L); Gal. *Loc. Aff.* III.9 (VIII 180,1–181,7 K). See Anastassiou and Irmer, 1997, volume II.2 p. 223.

It would have been better to make the causes those things whose excess in the body we can actually point out. His second error was that he did not even come close to the true cause of quotidian and tertian fevers. In quotidian fevers an excess of phlegm-like humour, which is wet and cold, is clearly evident; and in tertian fevers there is clearly an excess of yellow bile, this latter humour being, in its turn, extremely hot and dry. Therefore in the latter case the statement should have been that there is an excess of the element fire, and in quotidian fevers an excess of water; just as in quartan fevers the statement would be that the humour is black bile and the element is earth. Anyone who wished to learn in detail the nature of these fevers will find a full account in the treatises *On Crises* and *On the Different Kinds of Fevers*. It is not my habit to write the same things over and over about the same subjects; when I have given the scientific proof once or sometimes even twice, I then use the conclusion of the proof in my other books.[25]

We can see from this passage that Galen is criticising Plato for ignoring what Hippocrates has said about the causes of the different types of periodic fever. He sets up the argument against Plato by pointing out two significant errors in Plato's theory of the cause of the fevers. The first mistake relates to Plato's use of the four cosmic elements, rather than the four humours, to explain the cause of the different fevers in the body.[26] The second error is that Plato has

---

25 ἀμελῶς οὖν ἔσχε περί τε τὴν τῶν αὐτῶν τούτων ἐξέτασιν ἔτι τε μᾶλλον ὧν ἔγραψεν ὁ Ἱπποκράτης περὶ τῶν πλεοναζόντων νοσημάτων ἐν ἑκάστῃ τῶν ἡλικιῶν τε καὶ ὡρῶν, ὡς εἴ γε προσεσχήκει τὸν νοῦν αὐτοῖς, οὐκ ἂν ἐγεγράφει ταῦτα· "τὸ μὲν οὖν ἐκ πυρὸς ὑπερβολῆς μάλιστα νοσήσαν σῶμα συνεχῆ καύματα καὶ πυρετοὺς ἀπεργάζεται, τὸ δὲ ἐξ ἀέρος ἀφημερινούς, τριταίους δὲ ὕδατος διὰ τὸ νωθέστερον ἀέρος καὶ πυρὸς αὐτὸ εἶναι, τὸ δὲ γῆς τέταρτον ὂν νωθέστατον τούτων ἐν τετρα-πλασίαις περιόδοις χρόνου καθαιρόμενον τεταρταίους πυρετοὺς ποιῆσαν ἀπαλλάττεται μόλις." ἐν τούτῳ τῷ λόγῳ πρῶτον μὲν ἡμάρτηκε κατὰ τὰ κοινὰ στοιχεῖα ἁπάντων σωμάτων, οὐ κατὰ τὰ τῶν ἐναίμων ζῴων ποιησάμενος τὴν αἰτιολογίαν τῶν περιοδικῶν πυρετῶν· ἄμεινον γὰρ ἦν ἃ καὶ δεῖξαι δυνάμεθα κατὰ τὸ σῶμα πλεονάζοντα, ταῦτ' αἰτιᾶσθαι· δεύτερον δ' ὅτι τῶν ἀφημερι-νῶν καὶ τριταίων πυρετῶν οὐδ' ἐγγὺς ἧκε τῆς ἀληθοῦς αἰτίας. φαίνεται γὰρ ἐναργῶς ἐπὶ μὲν τῶν ἀφημερινῶν ὁ φλεγματώδης πλεονάζων χυμός, ὑγρὸς καὶ ψυχρὸς ὤν, ἐπὶ δὲ τῶν τριταίων ὁ τῆς ξανθῆς χολῆς, πάλιν αὖ καὶ οὗτος ἄκρως θερμὸς καὶ ξηρός· ὥστ' ἐπὶ τούτου μὲν ἐχρῆν εἰρῆσθαι πλεονάζειν τὸ τοῦ πυρὸς στοιχεῖον, ἐπ' ἀμφημερινοῦ δὲ τὸ τοῦ ὕδατος, ὥσπερ ἐν τοῖς τεταρταίοις χυμὸν μὲν τὴν μέλαιναν χολήν, στοιχεῖον δὲ τὴν γῆν. ὅστις δ' ἑκάστου τῶν εἰρημένων ἀκριβῶς ἐκμαθεῖν βούλεται τὴν φύσιν, ἔν τε τοῖς περὶ κρίσεων ὑπομνήμασι κἂν τοῖς περὶ τῆς διαφορᾶς τῶν πυρετῶν ἐξειργασμένον τὸν λόγον ἔχει. ἐγὼ δ' οὐκ εἴωθα πολλάκις ὑπὲρ τῶν αὐτῶν τὰ αὐτὰ γράφειν, ἀλλ' ἅπαξ ἢ καὶ δὶς ἐνίοτε τὴν ἀπόδειξιν εἰπὼν ἐν τοῖς ἄλλοις βιβλίοις τῷ συμπεράσματι τῆς ἀποδείξεως χρῶμαι· *PHP*, VIII.6.38–43, CMG 4,2,1, p. 520,3–26 De Lacy (v 697,5–698,16 κ), translation by De Lacy.

26 In *PHP* (VIII.5.4–7, CMG 4,2,1, p. 506,12–24 De Lacy (v 680,9–681,8 κ)), Galen criticised Plato

incorrectly assigned the qualities to the quotidian and tertian fevers. We find that Galen begins his criticism of Plato with reference to the writing of Hippocrates, but he ends the passage by citing his own works, *On Crises* and *On the Differences of Fevers*, for the best sources to understand the cause of the different types of fever. Thus Galen has cleverly included Hippocrates as the authority on this subject, but if anyone wants to learn about this topic they need to consult Galen's works, rather than Hippocratic treatises. It is true that Galen is clear about the association between black bile and quartan fever in the two texts that he cites. In *On Crises*, 'black bile' (μέλαινα χολή) is in excess (πλεονάζειν) when a person is suffering from quartan fever.[27] In this text, Galen also emphasises the importance of the uneven mix of the qualities 'cold and dry' with the characteristics of the autumn season. This is discussed in relation to his view that this fever will be more likely to be produced in those suffering from a melancholic condition, having a diet that promotes black bile in the body and where the quartan fever has become an epidemic.[28] We find in *On the Differences of Fevers* that quartan fever is more prevalent in those who are naturally more melancholic (μελαγχολικώτερα), which comes from the effect of the cold and dry (ξηρὰ καὶ ψυχρά) qualities, such as for those who are past the prime age of life and the conditions of autumn.[29] We also find that Galen refers to the quartan fevers in *On the Properties of Foodstuffs*. In this text, he calls the quartan fever a disease of those suffering from the conditions related to the 'melancholic humours' (μελαγχολικοὶ χυμοί), which includes diseases of the skin, such as cancer, elephantiasis, scabies and leprosy. Galen is warning against the intake of too much beef that is thick by anyone who has a melancholic constitution.[30] In his commentary on a passage from *Epidemics I*, Galen tells us that the production of the quartan fever cannot be explained simply by a particular condition (κατάστασις). Instead, this type of fever is caused by an increase in 'black bile' (μέλαινα χολή) in those who have a melancholic nature (μελαγχολικὴ φύσις), where the black bile has not been sufficiently evacuated.[31]

---

for not acknowledging the importance of the four humours for explanations of health and disease in the body. See Lloyd, 2008: 43.

27   *Cris.* II.3 (IX 652,12–14 K).
28   *Cris.* II.4 (IX 659,6–15 K). See Anastassiou and Irmer, 1997, volume II.2 p. 87.
29   *Diff. Feb.* II.1; II.5 (VII 335,10–15; 343,10–14 K).
30   *Alim. Fac.* III.1, CMG V 4,2, p. 333,1–7 Helmreich (VI 661,12–662,2 K). See Siegel, 1968: 285–299.
31   *Epid. I*, VI (II 620,10–622,2 L). Jones suggests that the Hippocratic physician was mistaken in thinking that there was an actual change of one type of fever to the quartan fever. He explains that in cases of malaria, there are many different illnesses mixed together and after time the quartan is left because it lasts a long time, this gives the impression that it

So far, the implication from Galen's writing is that an excess of forms of the natural black bile, rather than the altered type, are the cause of the quartan fevers.
There are also similar direct statements about the cause of quartan fever from
natural black bile in Galen's *Commentary on Aphorisms, On Tremor, Palpitation,
Spasm and Rigor*, and *Prognosis by Pulses*.[32] In all of these cases, we see that
Galen uses μέλαινα χολή and μελαγχολικὸς χυμός interchangeably in respect to
the physical substance that causes quartan fever. We have seen this many times
before, when Galen has used both of these terms to refer to different forms of
black bile.

We can see from the passage from *On the Doctrines of Hippocrates and Plato*
above (pages 136–137), that Galen accuses Plato of failing to read material on
Hippocrates' view on this subject. The question is which Hippocratic texts
should Plato have consulted in this case? Galen does not name them and only
refers to his own books when he recommends how the proper understanding of
quartan fevers should be obtained. However, Plato, who lived many centuries
before Galen, would clearly not have been able to read Galen's books and so,
would only have access to certain medical texts, such as those written by the
Hippocratic physicians. If we take Galen's first statement from *On the Doctrines
of Hippocrates and Plato*, he says that Plato should have consulted Hippocrates'
writing about the diseases that are produced in a particular time of life (ἡλικιῶν) or season (ὡρῶν). The Hippocratic *On the Nature of Man*, although not
named explicitly here, is an important work that Galen frequently refers to,
which does contain a section on quartan fevers and black bile:

> Therefore, you will know that the quartan fevers share in [the qualities]
> of black bile; of autumn mostly that the men are seized by the quartan
> fevers, between the ages of twenty-five and forty-five, this age is the most
> likely of all the ages, and autumn is the most likely of all the seasons, when
> a man is mastered by black bile.[33]

---

has been produced from the illnesses occurring earlier on, Jones, 1923a: 157 (note 1). Galen
provides his interpretation of this passage in his *Hipp. Epid.* (I.II.21, CMG V 10,1, p. 59,22–29
Wenkebach (XVIIa 114,14–115,6 K)).

32   *Hipp. Aph.* VII.40 (XVIIIa 143,5–14 K); *Trem. Palp.* 7 (VII 633,11–14 K); *Praes. Puls.* I.4 (IX 247,
18–248,2 K).

33   γνώσῃ δὲ τῷδε, ὅτι οἱ τεταρταῖοι πυρετοὶ μετέχουσι τοῦ μελαγχολικοῦ· φθινοπώρου μάλιστα οἱ
ἄνθρωποι ἁλίσκονται ὑπὸ τῶν τεταρταίων καὶ ἐν τῇ ἡλικίῃ τῇ ἀπὸ πέντε καὶ εἴκοσιν ἐτέων ἐς τὰ
πέντε καὶ τεσσαράκοντα, ἡ δὲ ἡλικίη αὕτη ὑπὸ μελαίνης χολῆς κατέχεται μάλιστα πασέων τῶν
ἡλικιῶν, ἥ τε φθινοπωρινὴ ὥρη μάλιστα πασέων τῶν ὡρέων. *Nat. Hom.* 15, CMG I 1,3, p. 204,14–
21 Jouanna (VI 68,8–14 L), adapted from a translation by Jones.

This passage provides all of the material that Galen needs to make his points about showing that Hippocrates had already identified black bile as being the basis of the cause of quartan fevers. We have the direct statement that quartan fevers come from black bile, but we also see that black bile is associated with both autumn and the age of life between twenty-five and forty-five. This would therefore be the perfect point of comparison that Galen could use to provide the evidence that Hippocrates is actually talking about black bile when he refers to the occurrence of quartan fevers in autumn and in people of a certain age in other treatises of the Hippocratic writings. However, there is a problem, as we find that Galen has rejected this whole section of *On the Nature of Man* because he does not believe it was written by Hippocrates. In his *Commentary on On the Nature of Man*, when Galen comes to the fifteenth section he objects firstly to the ordering of continuous, quotidian, tertian and quartan, as he says that in this passage the tertian fever comes to crisis after the quotidian fever. But this contradicts the writing of Hippocrates in *Epidemics* and *Aphorisms*, where the tertian fever is said to be the quickest to reach crisis. Another issue raised by Galen is that he is unhappy with the use of σύνοχος for 'continuous', as this is a more recent term and was not used by Hippocrates.[34] Galen's position against this passage is so strong that he condemns the writer of this section as a liar:

> So the man who has written these things was either such a sophist, or a quack, as seems likely, having appended this lie so that blame might be inflicted on the ancient author.[35]

The absence of any positive commentary or reference to this passage here, or any of Galen's other writing that has survived, does impact on the way that he can support his view that Hippocrates intended the explanation of the cause of quartan fevers to be an excess of black bile in the body. So, instead of *On the Nature of Man*, we find that Galen uses other Hippocratic works to present Hippocrates' view of the cause of quartan fevers.

There is a short passage in *Koan Prognoses* that informs us that quartan fevers are more likely to be produced from fevers that are more irregular in period, especially in the autumn and are more likely to be suffered by peo-

---

34   See chapter 2, section 3 above for more information about Galen's rejection of this part of *On the Nature of Man*.

35   ὥσθ' ὁ ταῦτα γράψας ἢ τοιοῦτος ἦν σοφιστὴς ἢ πανοῦργος ἄνθρωπος, ὡς ἔοικεν, παρεγγράψας τὸ ψεῦδος ἕνεκα τοῦ προστρίψασθαι ψόγον τῷ παλαιῷ. *HNH*, II.22, CMG V 9,1, p. 88,4–7 Mewaldt (XV 172,11–14 K), adapted from a translation by Lewis.

ple over the age of thirty.[36] We know that Galen did acknowledge that some parts of *Koan Prognoses* were of the standard that he expects from a genuine work by Hippocrates, so Galen may be referring to this work.[37] However, since Galen does not mention the information regarding the season and time of life, which we find in the passage from *Koan Prognoses*, it is difficult to identify this text as the Hippocratic source to which Galen refers. Another substantial passage from *On Diseases II* contains a lot of information about the conditions that bring about quartan fevers and the best way to treat this type of illness. In this text we find that quartan fevers are suffered by those 'in an unclean state from another disease' (ἐξ ἄλλης νούσου ... ἀκάθαρτον). The recommendation is to cleanse the body 'downwards' (κάτω), which could imply that excess bile needs to be removed. The presence of too much bile could also be inferred by the use of 'white hellebore' (λευκός ἐλλέβορος), as part of the many different substances recommended as treatments for quartan fever in this passage.[38] We have seen earlier that it is possible that Galen has used material from *On Diseases II* in relation to his characterisation of the properties of altered black bile. However, in this case there is no such evidence to suggest he intended *On Diseases II* to be used by Plato to understand Hippocrates' view on quartan fevers.[39] In contrast to these two examples, Galen does discuss the content of a passage from the Hippocratic *Aphorisms* (III.22) that contains a reference to the quartan fevers that occur as a summer and autumn disease, alongside a list of diseases, which includes disease of the spleen and melancholia.[40] We find the following interpretation of this aphorism in Galen's *Commentary on Aphorisms*:

> Moreover, he [Hippocrates] says of quartan fevers that they are produced in this season, obviously being caused by black bile, which has two types of production, one from the over-heating of yellow bile, and the other from the thick blood.[41]

---

36   *Coac.* 139 (V 612,16–18 L). There are also other examples of quartan fevers in *Aer.* (VII (II 28,4–8 L)) and *Epid. I* (XXVI (II 680,9–682,2 L)), but these only mention the fever without any detail about its production.

37   See chapter 2, section 3 above.

38   *Morb. II*, XLIII (VII 60,6–24 L). Hellebore was used as a purgative drug for both types of bile, yellow or black. For example, see *Epid. V*, II; LXXX (V 204,8–9; 250,5 L).

39   See chapter 2, section 3 above.

40   *Aph.* III.22 (IV 496,4–8 L).

41   καὶ μέντοι καὶ τεταρταίους πυρετοὺς ἐν ταύτῃ τῇ ὥρᾳ γίγνεσθαί φησιν, ἐπὶ τῇ μελαίνῃ δηλονότι συνισταμένους χολῇ, διττὴν ἐχούσῃ τὴν γένεσιν, ἐκ μὲν τῆς ξανθῆς ὑπεροπτηθείσης τὴν ἑτέραν, ἐκ δὲ τοῦ παχέος αἵματος τὴν ἑτέραν. *Hipp. Aph.* III.22 (XVIIb 622,2–6 K). Galen also refers to this passage in an earlier part of this commentary, but does not give any further detail (III.5 (XVIIb 570,7–571,6 K)). See Anastassiou and Irmer, 1997, volume II.1 p. 103.

Here we have Galen explaining how Hippocrates can write about the occurrence of quartan fevers in both summer and autumn.[42] In autumn the cause of quartan fevers is easily explained, as in this season the natural black bile humour increases in the body and so there is more susceptibility for people to suffer from illness related to black bile. However, in summer the situation is more complicated, as there is not a large amount of natural black bile in the body in this season. But, we have already discovered the reason why diseases related to black bile can occur in the summer, as the heat causes altered black bile to be produced by the 'roasting' of the humours in the body.[43] Therefore, the large amount of yellow bile present in the body in summer can change into altered black bile under the conditions of intense heating. We have seen that he refers to natural forms of black bile as the cause of quartan fevers, with no mention of altered black bile. However, Galen now needs to explain why there is a passage, in one of his 'favoured' Hippocratic texts, which has quartan fevers occurring in summer, the 'hot and dry' season. Galen uses his theory on the production of altered black bile in conditions that are 'hot and dry' to explain this aphorism. However, he does not say whether there are differences between the quartan fevers produced in summer or autumn and if the acidic properties of the altered black bile cause additional complications for the suffering of the patient.

Galen provides more information on the cause of different fevers in the different seasons in his comments on the following passage from the Hippocratic *Prognostic*:

> If the fever be continuous you must expect the abscession to be of this type, but the disease will resolve into a quartan if it intermit and attack in an irregular fashion, and if autumn approach while it acts in this way. Just as the abscessions occur when the patients are under thirty, so the quartans supervene more often when they are thirty or over.[44]

---

42   Galen is presenting his interpretation of a passage from *Aph.* (III.22 (IV 496,4–8 L)), which discusses the types of diseases that occur in autumn and summer.

43   See chapter 4, section 2 above.

44   χρὴ δὲ τὴν μὲν τοιαύτην ἀπόστασιν προσδέχεσθαι συνεχέος ἐόντος τοῦ πυρετοῦ, ἐς δὲ τεταρταῖον καταστήσεσθαι, ἢν διαλείπῃ τε καὶ ἐπιλαμβάνῃ πεπλανημένον τρόπον καὶ ταῦτα ποιέων τῷ φθινοπώρῳ πελάσῃ. ὥσπερ δὲ τοῖσι νεωτέροισι τριάκοντα ἐτέων αἱ ἀποστάσιες γίνονται, οὕτως οἱ τεταρταῖοι μᾶλλον τοῖσι τριακονταέτεσι καὶ γεραιτέροισι. *Prog.* XXIV, II 182,1–7 L, translation by Jones. Galen also quotes this passage as part of a longer section in his *Cris.* (III.11 (IX 753,8–754,10 K)), where he is reporting what Hippocrates has said on the different types of fever. See Anastassiou and Irmer, 1997, volume II.2 pp. 131–135.

In his *Commentary on Prognostic*, Galen begins his interpretation of this passage by reporting that he has discussed the association between the quartan fevers and the 'melancholic humours' (μελαγχολικοὶ χυμοί) in another of his works called *On the Differences of Fevers*. In this way, Galen is repeating what he said in the passage from *On the Doctrines of Hippocrates and Plato* (see pages 136–137 above). This is because he wants to make this association between black bile and the quartan fevers clear, as it does not appear in the passage from *Prognostic*.[45] However, in *Commentary on Prognostic*, Galen tells us that there is an extreme heating of the humours in those with continuous fevers in the summer. The body may be able to cope with the increase of black bile in the body, as long as it can be voided as quickly as possible. However, this is more difficult for older people (ἐν ταῖς ἡλικίαις ἡ παρακμή and ἄχρι τοῦ γήρως) and in autumn, where the cold inhibits the evacuation of black bile from the body.[46] Here, there is some ambiguity caused by Galen's tendency not to provide different names for the different types of black bile. The reference to the heating of the humours suggests that the altered black bile is being produced, but the case of the evacuation of black bile in autumn due to the cold indicates the natural form of this humour. However, we can resolve this by taking into account the process that altered black bile can be restored to its natural qualities by a cooling effect that occurs when the heat is removed. Therefore, large amounts of altered black bile are produced from the heating of the humours, but the cooling process means that it changes back to the 'cold and dry' form of natural black bile that is difficult to remove from the body in autumn. In this way, Galen can select passages from *Prognostic* and *Aphorisms*, which he considers to be superior Hippocratic works, to show that Hippocrates is in agreement with this characterisation of the effect of black bile to cause quartan fevers.

Therefore, all that is left for Galen is to base his argument for Hippocrates' agreement with his own theory about black bile causing quartan fevers on the following Hippocratic texts: the combination of a reading of *Prognostic* and the earlier sections of *On the Nature of Man*, along with supporting material from *Aphorisms*. However, despite Galen's rejection of the fifteenth section of *On the Nature of Man*, I think that this is an important source for Galen in *On the Doctrines of Hippocrates and Plato*. But Galen is unable to quote this part directly, as this would contradict his rejection of it. We have seen already that Galen tells us that in *On the Doctrines of Hippocrates and Plato* he is avoiding quoting from *On the Nature of Man*, as he suggests that he has covered all the material worth

---

45   In fact, black bile is not referred to at all in the *Prognostic*, see chapter 2, section 3 above.

46   *Hipp. Prog.* III.32–33, CMG V 9,2, pp. 355,23–358,8 Heeg (XVIIIb 277,14–283,2 K).

noting in *On the Elements According to Hippocrates*. Therefore, Galen uses the type of information found in the fifteenth section of *On the Nature of Man* and paraphrases it so that he does not need to cite it. The problem is that Galen suspects that this part of *On the Nature of Man* is a Hellenistic forgery and so on this basis, it probably would not have been written until after Plato's death. It is difficult to identify any particular Hippocratic text, apart from the passage in the fifteenth section of *On the Nature of Man*, which Plato could have read to understand the Hippocratic humoral system for the production of quartan fevers from black bile, rather than the cosmic elemental earth. Therefore, it is unclear whether Plato would have been able to draw such conclusions relating to quartan fevers and black bile and even Galen himself recommends his own texts as the best way to understand the relationship between them.

3   Cases Where the Presence of Black Bile Indicates a Terminal
       Disease

Moving on from these specific cases of melancholy and the quartan fevers, I now want to discuss the more general diseases that Galen attributes to black bile. In the earlier section about diseases of the spleen, I discussed Galen's quotation of a passage from the Hippocratic *Aphorisms* in his treatise *On the Natural Faculties*.[47] This is part of Galen's argument for the teleological basis of the design of the spleen to remove a potentially harmful substance from the body. The passage from the Hippocratic *Aphorisms* (IV.24) that Galen uses is important, as he refers to it in some of his other works. For example, in *On the Utility of the Parts*, Galen uses this aphorism when he discusses the situation where black bile must be quickly removed from the body. Here Galen is refer-ring to the altered form of black bile, as it causes severe ulceration when it is present in the body, which is not the case for natural forms of black bile. We are told that the sensitivity of the bowels causes an immediate action to remove the altered black bile. The shorter the time that this substance is in the body, the less harm it can do. Unfortunately, the long and winding structure of the intestines allows the altered black bile time to cause severe ulceration.[48] Galen provides a similar explanation in *On Black Bile*:

---

47   See chapter 6, section 4 above.
48   *UP*, V.10 (III 381,6–382,5 K). See also *Hipp. Aph.* IV.24 (XVIIb 688,8–689,4 K).

From the same indications that it is in fact possible to recognise for certain the effective cause, it is clearly evident that both yellow bile and black bile corrode one of the intestines or the other at different times, wherever it is especially established, and after a certain time, they make dysentery incurable. On account of this Hippocrates wrote in *Aphorisms*: "Dysentery, if it begins from black bile, is fatal." I said before that everything that is ulcerated on account of black bile is incurable, unless you want to term as healing the excision of the whole of the affected part, which is cutting round in a circle up to the parts that are unaffected.[49]

We see in this passage that Galen is referring to the altered black bile, as this type of ulceration comes from its harmful acidic properties. This is emphasised in Galen's comparison of the two types of dysentery caused by yellow bile and altered black bile. He explains that altered black bile causes more severe ulceration because of viscosity, as it is a thicker substance than yellow bile and therefore moves more slowly through the body. This altered black bile has such an effect on the body that the condition will be incurable compared to the effect of yellow bile. Galen has been able to support his theory of the terminal effect of ulceration by altered black bile with reference to an aphorism, which he attributes to Hippocrates. We saw earlier that Galen attempts to emphasise the importance of this aphorism in relation to another one, as he believes they are in conflict with each other. However, Galen is mistaken because there is no such contradiction.[50] But, Galen wants to highlight this aphorism as an example of Hippocrates' agreement with his overall argument for the importance of black bile and the spleen to understand health and disease in the body. In this way Galen wants to use Hippocrates, as the originator of this type of theory, in his polemic against the followers of Erasistratus.

But it is not just dysentery, associated with the presence of the altered black bile, which is considered deadly. What we can see from the passage above in *On Black Bile* is that Galen extends this fatal prognosis from dysentery to all ulcerations caused by altered black bile. He tells us that 'everything that is ulcerated

---

49 ἐφ' ὧν γοῦν οἷόν τέ ἐστι βεβαίως διαγνῶναι τὴν ἐργασαμένην αἰτίαν, ἐναργῶς ἐπὶ τούτων φαίνεται καὶ ξανθὴ καὶ μέλαινα χολὴ διαβιβρώσκουσαι τῶν ἐντέρων ἄλλοτε ἄλλο, καθ' ὅτιπερ ἂν μάλιστα στηριχθῶσιν, καί ποτε καὶ τελέως ἀνίατον ἐργαζόμεναι τὴν δυσεντερίαν. καὶ διὰ τοῦτο Ἱπποκράτης ἐν Ἀφορισμοῖς ἔγραψε· "Δυσεντερίη, ἢν ἀπὸ χολῆς μελαίνης ἄρξηται, θανάσιμον." ἐγὼ δὲ πρόσθεν εἶπον ἀνίατα πάντα εἶναι τὰ διὰ μέλαιναν χολὴν ἑλκωθέντα, πλὴν εἴ τις ἴασιν ἐθέλει καλεῖν, ὅταν ἐκκόψῃ τὸ πεπονθὸς μόριον ὅλον ἐν κύκλῳ περιτεμὼν ἄχρι τῶν ἀπαθῶν. At. Bil. 5, CMG V 4,1,1, p. 80,7–15 De Boer (V 122,2–12 K), adapted from a translation by Grant. See Anastassiou and Irmer, 1997, volume II.2 p. 90.

50 See chapter 6, section 4 above.

because of black bile is incurable' (ἀνίατα πάντα εἶναι τὰ διὰ μέλαιναν χολὴν ἑλκω-θέντα). This shows that Galen believed that any ulceration of altered black bile would lead to the death of the patient. This statement is made after the quotation from *Aphorisms* and this could imply that Galen considers Hippocrates to have the same opinion regarding the terminal prognosis of altered black bile ulcerating the body in this way. In fact, there is another passage from *Aphorisms* that does imply that the presence of black bile should be taken as a general sign of a terminal case:

> Should black bile be evacuated at the beginning of any disease, whether upwards or downwards, it is a mortal symptom.[51]

Galen provides more detail in his interpretation of this aphorism in his *Commentary on Aphorisms*. He tells us that this condition indicates that the vital organs inside of the body (σπλάγχνον) have been affected by 'black bile' (μέλαινα χολή) to such an extent that death will normally follow. This is part of the importance of observation that Galen recommends to physicians, as the diagnosis of an illness can be determined by the type of waste matter that is evacuated from the body at certain critical times (καιρός).[52] In this case, Galen's decision to avoid precise naming of the different types of black bile makes it more difficult to determine which form of black bile he is discussing here. However, in this case the terminal illness implies that it is the altered form of black bile that is present. But Galen needs to use μέλαινα χολή, as this is used by the author of the Hippocratic *Aphorisms*.

The reason for Galen's focus on black bile comes from his view that the presence of this humour in evacuated matter can indicate the fatal nature of a disease. The support for this theory is strengthened by yet another passage from the Hippocratic Aphorisms:

> When patients have become reduced through disease, acute or chronic, or through wounds or through any other cause, a discharge of black bile, or as it were of black blood, means death on the following day.[53]

---

51 Νοσημάτων ὁκόσων ἀρχομένων, ἢν χολὴ μέλαινα ἢ ἄνω ἢ κάτω ὑπέλθῃ, θανάσιμον. *Aph.* IV.22 (IV 510,3–4 L), translation by Jones.

52 *Hipp. Aph.* IV.21 (XVIIb 683,10–684,14 K). See Anastassiou and Irmer, 1997, volume II.1 p. 112. Galen also quotes this passage in *Cris.* (I.6 (IX 571,15–572,2 K)). See Anastassiou and Irmer, 1997, volume II.2 pp. 155–156. We also find both Hippocratic passages, the reference to fatal black bile dysentery and any disease beginning with black bile, quoted by Galen in *Diff. Resp.* (III.9 (VII 935,1–11 K)). See Anastassiou and Irmer, 1997, volume II.2 pp. 167–171.

53 Ὁκόσοισιν ἐκ νοσημάτων ὀξέων ἢ πολυχρονίων, ἢ ἐκ τραυμάτων, ἢ ἄλλως λελεπτυσμένοισι χολὴ

This is the next aphorism, after the one quoted above, but this time black blood (αἷμα μέλαν) is identified in addition to μέλαινα χολή. In his commentary on this passage, Galen explains that this aphorism is required as an addition to the previous aphorism, as it is necessary to distinguish between what is truly black bile and what only looks like black bile. In this case, the comparison is between black blood and the altered form of black bile. Therefore, Galen is implying that Hippocrates is referring to the altered black bile in this passage from the *Aphorisms*. He goes so far as to say that Hippocrates 'showed clearly to us that we were right to distinguish black bile from the general black substances' (ἐδήλωσε δὲ καὶ ὅτι καλῶς ἡμεῖς διωρίσαμεν ἀπὸ τῶν μελάνων τὴν μέλαιναν χολήν).[54] Therefore, on the basis of a few lines from the Hippocratic *Aphorisms*, Galen has supported his presentation of the altered black bile with the authority of Hippocrates. This is his strategy in *On the Natural Faculties* and *On Black Bile* that he uses to attack and refute the ideas of the followers of Asclepiades and Erasistratus by deploying past authorities, such as Hippocrates, even when the actual evidence cannot be easily found directly in their writing.

4   Summary

We can see from Galen's writing that both the non-ideal natural black bile and altered black bile are important for his explanation of various diseases caused by this humour. When it comes to the illness known as melancholy, Galen is careful to identify non-ideal natural black bile, which he calls the thick, melancholic humour, as being responsible for this disease, rather than the ideal natural or altered forms of black bile. Galen needs to make this distinction between his three main types of black bile, as he does not want to associate the ideal natural black bile with this illness, as he presents this form as beneficial to our health. Further to this, in Galen's medical view, the condition of melancholy is treatable and this is why Galen does not want to implicate the altered forms of black bile, as they could ulcerate the brain making the condition incurable. Galen also does not apply such a strict nomenclature to explain the cause of the quartan fevers from different types of black bile. We find that both terms for black bile are used by Galen in association with quartan fevers. Further to this we also find that the altered form of black bile is identified by Galen as another cause of quartan fevers. If we investigate diseases caused by black bile in the

---

μέλαινα ἢ ὁκοῖον αἷμα μέλαν ὑπέλθῃ, τῇ ὑστεραίῃ ἀποθνῄσκουσιν. *Aph.* IV.23 (IV 510,5–8 L), translation by Jones.

54   *Hipp. Aph.* XVIIb 687,1–688,3 K. See Anastassiou and Irmer, 1997, volume II.1 p. 111.

Galenic Corpus more generally, we find that altered black bile in the body is often fatal. We can see that parts of the Hippocratic *Aphorisms* have been used by Galen to show that Hippocrates had already warned of the deadly effect of black bile in the body. The importance of this aphorism is elevated further by Galen's rejection of another passage in *Aphorisms*, which he believes contradicts it. In this way, Galen can select and manipulate various treatises from past authorities, which he can use to support his own theory on the effect of black bile on the body.

CHAPTER 8

Conclusion

My analysis of the way that Galen uses 'black bile' for his explanation of health and disease in the body shows that it is important to understand the context of the particular treatise, or even section of a treatise, concerned. Therefore, it is very difficult, if not impossible, to summarise Galen's 'theory of black bile' on the basis of a single comprehensive framework. This is because Galen does not apply a consistent theory of black bile in his writing, sometimes it is one substance with different characteristics, at other times it is described as completely different substances, even with different names. A large amount of modern scholarship has either attempted to explain or resolve inconsistencies in Galen's writing on black bile or has tried to ignore them. However, this approach will not allow us to fully understand the way that Galen has characterised black bile, as these very inconsistencies are essential to provide key information concerning Galen's strategy in developing a theory of black bile, and refute his rivals' arguments on the importance of black bile in medicine. The main factor causing Galen difficulty in maintaining consistency between his treatises, and even within them, is his attempt to represent Hippocrates as the founder and originator of a biological theory based on qualities, elements and humours, which was adopted and developed by a number of philosophers and physicians over several centuries. This means that Galen not only needs to show agreement on black bile between Hippocrates and other authorities such as Plato, Aristotle, Diocles and Praxagoras, but he also faces significant problems in showing that there is consistency between the texts of the Hippocratic writings on black bile. This task to obtain agreement between such a wide range of sources is very difficult in the case of the black bile humour, as the evidence that we have suggests that this substance was either considered as an insignificant residue or even completely ignored in the majority of ancient medical theories.

One way that Galen tries to overcome such issues is to present black bile as three main types, which I have called: ideal natural, non-ideal natural and altered black bile. These distinct definitions of black bile represent the most important characteristics of this type of humour in relation to health and disease in the body. What we find is that Galen's characterisation of the physical structure and function of black bile is his own creation, as it does not exist, in the way that Galen defines it, in any medical theory produced before him. We have seen that this division of black bile into three main types is required

© KONINKLIJKE BRILL NV, LEIDEN, 2019 | DOI:10.1163/9789004382794_010

as he tries to show agreement between the many and varied sources such as the different treatises in the Hippocratic writings, philosophical works by Plato and Aristotle, along with the medical theories produced by physicians like Diocles, Praxagoras and Rufus of Ephesus. However, Galen presents his theory of black bile as if he is just providing more detailed information and an enhanced explanation that appears within Hippocrates' writing and is continued by certain philosophers and physicians afterwards. It is significant that Galen does not boast that he has created a new theory of black bile to challenge the views of his rivals, but instead he wants to present this theory with support from Hippocrates and other prominent authorities on medicine. It is more important to Galen that he is able to draw upon material from a wide range of sources to strengthen his arguments concerning the physical description and function of black bile, even when no such evidence can be found in the sources to which he refers.

We have seen that Galen uses the treatises from Dioscurides' list of the most genuine Hippocratic texts: *Aphorisms, Prognostic, On Regimen in Acute Diseases, Airs, Waters and Places,* and *Epidemics I* and *III,* to support his characterisation of black bile. However, Galen also includes the first eight chapters of *On the Nature of Man* as a key Hippocratic text on black bile. But there is no evidence that any other physician, philosopher, or commentator had regarded the first part of *On the Nature of Man* as meriting this attribution to Hippocrates himself. In fact, we can see from the references by Aristotle that this treatise was generally acknowledged to be by Polybos. The evidence suggests that the four-humour system in this treatise was not as highly regarded as Galen makes it out to be in the other Hippocratic works and the medical writing of some of the philosophers and physicians who came afterwards. Galen's particular emphasis on this treatise and its humoral theory has had a major impact on modern scholarship, as there is a tendency to regard the four-humour system of *On the Nature of Man* as having a more significant role in Galen's characterisation of black bile than it actually does. In fact, this is what Galen would want us to believe, as he makes a large number of claims about the work of Hippocrates on black bile that cannot be substantiated from the ideas contained in *On the Nature of Man* alone. This is because the content on black bile in this treatise only provides Galen with information that he associates with the ideal natural form of black bile, which is essential for maintaining the humoral balance for health. But, this text does not contain any information for his characterisation of the non-ideal natural and altered forms of black bile. Therefore, Galen's attempt to show that *On the Nature of Man* is an essential reference work for information on the non-ideal natural and altered forms of black bile is inconsistent with the actual content of this Hippocratic treatise. But Galen's strategy is to convince his audience that Hippocrates did intend these other forms of black bile to be interpreted as the cause of certain types of disease and that the spleen is designed to remove unwanted black bile from the body. An example of Galen's strategy can be found in *On the Natural Faculties*, where Galen explicitly names *On the Nature of Man* as a text that should be read by Erasistratus for key information relating to Hippocrates' superior teleological theory and specifically on the association between black bile and the spleen. However, I have shown that there is no such material that provides the level of detail on the function of the spleen to remove non-ideal natural black bile in *On the Nature of Man*.

When it comes to analysing Galen's writing on black bile more generally, some modern scholars, such as Jacques Jouanna, have attempted to provide a resolution to perceived inconsistencies between Galen's characterisation of black bile, such as in *On the Natural Faculties* and *On Black Bile*, based on the pairing of 'cold and dry' qualities in order to show that Galen's overall aim was to be consistent with the ideas contained in *On the Nature of Man*. However, my analysis undermines this argument, as Galen is not always striving to reconcile the different forms of black bile in relation to the 'cold and dry' qualitative definition of black bile found in *On the Nature of Man*. Instead, although Galen acknowledges the importance of the four-humour system of this treatise, he is more interested in providing material on black bile that meets his own criteria for sound theoretical arguments that is consistent with any historical or current empirical information on black bile that he wants to use. Therefore, the description of black bile in *On the Nature of Man* is only a part of the information that Galen can utilise to argue his position against his rivals. It is more important that he has a flexible theory that takes information from a wide range of sources so that he can argue against the rival theories of the followers of Erasistratus and Asclepiades.

We have seen that it was important for Galen's theory of black bile to draw upon the material from various treatises in the Hippocratic writings. There is evidence that Galen wants to show that the texts from Dioscurides' list of the best examples of Hippocrates' works are in agreement with Galen's characterisation of the different types of black bile. All these texts are used by Galen in some way to support his view of black bile, but some are more prominent than others, particularly in cases where he wants to quote a Hippocratic source. We find that *Aphorisms* is frequently used by Galen to support his work on black bile, which is a text that contains a large amount of material on black bile in different contexts. This is in contrast to the *Prognostic* and *Epidemics I* and *III* that do not refer to black bile by name, but contain some references to black matter found in various waste substances evacuated from the body. However, the lack of reference to physical black bile does not stop Galen from interpreting these treatises as if 'Hippocrates' was in agreement with Galen's view of black bile in its different forms. In some cases there is more relevant information in other Hippocratic treatises, which Galen also considered authentic, such as *Koan Prognoses* and *On Humours*. But we generally find that he ignores this material in favour of what he considers to be the 'best and most genuine' Hippocratic works. Further to this, it appears that he is not always consistent with his own concept of authenticity of Hippocratic works. I have identified possible examples within Galen's writing on black bile where he may have chosen to make reference to certain treatises, as if they were written by Hippocrates, which in other places in his writing appear to have been rejected as inauthentic by him. For example, it is possible that Galen has glossed a passage from *On Diseases II*, which is a treatise that he does not consider to be written by Hippocrates, or one of his followers. However, this passage contains material that characterises a substance, which is acidic, harmful to the body, and effervesces in contact with the ground. This is similar to the way that Galen describes the properties of altered black bile. Another example of this strategy is where Galen may have paraphrased a passage from *On Places in Man*, which associates a disease of the spleen in relation to the swelling of the whole body, which Galen attributes to Hippocrates. I believe that it is likely that he is referring to this treatise in *On the Natural Faculties*. The problem is that Galen has denied elsewhere that *On Places in Man* is Hippocratic and so it may be the case that he is attempting to persuade his audience that this particular passage is from an authentic Hippocratic treatise. The reason is that in *On the Natural Faculties* he wants to show that there is agreement between Hippocrates and Plato on black bile and the spleen, which supports his overall aim in *On the Doctrines of Hippocrates and Plato*. This leads to the possibility that there is sometimes an inconsistency between what Galen identifies as an authentic Hippocratic treatise and what he references in practice, which he believes is necessary to provide the evidence to support his theory of black bile. Therefore, it is more important for him to demonstrate that there is evidence in a 'Hippocratic' source to support his argument from authority than his more general statements about authenticity of texts from the Hippocratic writings.

There are also important sources outside of the Hippocratic writings that Galen uses to support his work on black bile. It was important to Galen that Hippocrates had a similar approach to the idea of causation to Plato and Aristotle, as Galen wants to defend the very existence of black bile as an essential substance that explains health and disease in the body against the views of his main rivals. Galen wants to use the authority of Hippocrates, alongside that of Plato and Aristotle, when he wants to refute the views of Asclepiades and

Erasistratus on the basis of teleology. However, in contrast to the work of Plato and Aristotle, it is difficult to find a Hippocratic source that can provide the kind of teleological system that Galen attributes to Hippocrates. But it is important to Galen that Hippocrates is viewed as a teleological authority on par with these eminent philosophers. In addition, we also find that when Galen criticises Erasistratus on his question over the teleological status of bile and the spleen, Galen does not refer to Aristotle's similar stance on this topic. In this way, Galen brings together the authority of Hippocrates, Plato and Aristotle to justify the status of black bile as a fundamental substance and that the spleen is specifically designed to remove this humour from the body.

This methodology that brings together the material on black bile from a wide range of sources such as the Hippocratic writings, philosophy and other medical treatises, has made it very difficult for Galen to present black bile as a single substance based on a comprehensive and unified theory. This is the reason why he states that the three types of black bile are distinct in *On Affected Parts* because it is important for his explanation of the cause of melancholy by the non-ideal natural black bile. This is because he does not want to associate the cause of melancholy with the ideal natural and altered forms of black bile. We also find the same type of precise definition of the three kinds of black bile when Galen shows that the spleen is responsible for removing the non-ideal natural black bile from the blood. This approach is consistent within the context of the passages in some of his works, but most of the time we find that Galen cannot be so precise in his distinction between the different kinds of black bile. For example, when he defends the existence of black bile against the theories of Asclepiades and Erasistratus in *On the Natural Faculties* he uses the term 'black bile' (μέλαινα χολή), and not 'melancholic humour' (μελαγχολικὸς χυμός), to describe it both as a beneficial humour (ideal natural black bile) and as a harmful and potentially deadly substance in the body (non-ideal natural and altered forms of black bile). If Galen made such a distinction here it would weaken his argument and allow his critics to say that these are just different types of substances. They may say there is a form of black bile that exists as a residue in the body, but is not defined as a fundamental substance, such as a humour like blood or phlegm. But, Galen needs to support his case for black bile both as a fundamental humour and as a pathogenic substance that causes different types of disease, some that are potentially life threatening. What we find is that Galen often prefers to be 'loose', rather than 'precise', with his terminology for black bile, as it allows him to use different terms, or even just descriptions of substances, to characterise black bile in various ways. However, this sometimes creates inconsistency in many of his references to the different forms of black bile.

Therefore, when we read different Galenic treatises that contain information relating to black bile it is important that we understand the particular type of black bile that Galen is discussing in the context of the section of the treatise. In the case of *On the Elements According to Hippocrates* and *On the Doctrines of Hippocrates and Plato*, 'black bile' (μέλαινα χολή) should be understood on the basis of the ideal natural form, which has the characteristics of the black bile in the Hippocratic *On the Nature of Man*. This is the case for the majority of *Commentary on On the Nature of Man*. But care must be taken in this text, as we can also find one reference to 'melancholic humour' (μελαγχολικός χυμός), which is not used by Galen for ideal natural black bile. In this case, μελαγχολικός χυμός is the non-ideal natural black bile, which is similar to the description of this substance in the section on melancholy in *On Affected Parts*. There is a similar situation in *On the Utility of the Parts* and *On the Natural Faculties*, where the most common term is μέλαινα χολή with just one reference to μελαγχολικός χυμός in each text. In both of these cases Galen is referring to the substance that is drawn out of the blood by the spleen where he has decided to be more precise with his terminology for non-ideal natural black bile. However, it is more useful in these two texts for Galen to be less precise in his distinction between the three forms of black bile when he is attacking the views of rivals, such as Erasistratus, Asclepiades and their followers. This is because the collective naming of the three forms of black bile means that Galen can be more flexible with the material that he uses to characterise black bile when he wants to justify its importance in medicine. We can find a similar polemic against Erasistratus and his followers in *On Black Bile*, but this time Galen uses μελαγχολικός χυμός much more than μέλαινα χολή. However the difference between this treatise and *On the Natural Faculties* is that *On Black Bile* contains a large amount of material on the function of different types of black bile, mostly the altered forms, to explain the cause of different diseases and how these kinds of black bile can be correctly identified in waste matter evacuated from the body. Apart from a brief statement near the start of this treatise, the ideal natural black bile is not part of the overall discussion, as Galen focuses on the cause of disease and observation for diagnosis and prognosis. However, he does not differentiate by name between non-ideal natural and altered forms of black bile. He admits that he calls them both μελαγχολικός χυμός, but justifies it because he understands the important differences between these two types of black bile and so does not need to use different names to distinguish between them. The situation is even more complex in *On Mixtures*, as there are references to forms of black bile described as like sediment or as a substance produced from combustion. However, Galen only uses the term μέλαινα χολή and does not refer to μελαγχολικός χυμός at all. It is possible that Galen is using his language more 'loosely' here because he is not explaining the cause of a disease in detail and he wants to show agreement between Hippocrates and Aristotle on the importance of the qualities in medicine. In this case, it would be easier for Galen to refer to the different forms of black bile collectively, which would be consistent with the concept of a single form of black bile in the Hippocratic *On the Nature of Man* and material on black bile in Aristotelian works. Therefore, Galen will sometimes be precise with his naming of different types of black bile, but it is more convenient for him to use μέλαινα χολή for all three in these texts, with the occasional use of the term μελαγχολικὸς χυμός when he wants to be precise about a particular form of black bile. This is the basis of his overall strategy, as it is better that he is more flexible and can refer to black bile in different ways so that he can bring certain sources together, Hippocratic, Platonic, Aristotelian and many others, to show agreement and to support his arguments against rivals such as Asclepiades and Erasistratus.

Bibliography

Electronic Sources

Brockmann, C. (Dir.), *Corpus Medicorum Graecae/Latinorum*, last accessed 12th July 2016. cmg.bbaw.de/epubl/online/editionen.html

Henderson, J. (ed.), *Loeb Classical Library*, (1911), last accessed 12th July 2016. https://www.loebclassics.com/

Lewis, W.J. (trans.), 'Galen On Hippocrates' On the Nature of Man', *Medicina Antiqua*, UCL, last accessed 12th July 2016. http://www.ucl.ac.uk/~ucgajpd/medicina%20antiqua/tr_GNatHom.html

Pantelia, M. (Dir.), *Thesaurus Linguae Graecae*, (1972), last accessed 12th July 2016. http://stephanus.tlg.uci.edu/

Editions, Collections and Translations of Primary Sources

Anastassiou, A. and Irmer, D. (1997), *Testimonien zum Corpus Hippocraticum, II.1 und 2*, Vandenhoeck and Ruprecht, Göttingen.

Barras, V., Birchler, T. and Morand, A.-F. (1998), *Galien. De la bile noire*, Gallimard, Paris.

Bertier, J. (1972), *Mnesithée et Dieuchès*, Leiden.

Brock, A.J. (trans.) (1916), *Galen: On the Natural Faculties*, Cambridge, Massachusetts.

Bury, R.G. (trans.) (1929), *Plato: Timaeus, Critias, Cleitophon, Menexenus, Epistles*, Loeb, Cambridge, Massachusetts.

Craik, E.M. (trans.) (1998) *Hippocrates, Places in Man*, Oxford: Clarendon Press.

De Boer, W. (ed.) (1937a), *Galeni: De Atra Bile*, Akademie Verlag, Berlin.

De Boer, W. (ed.) (1937b), *Galeni: De Animi Cuiuslibet Peccatorum Dignotione et Curatione*, Akademie Verlag, Berlin.

De Lacy, P. (trans.) (1980), *Galen: On the Doctrines of Hippocrates and Plato*, Akademie Verlag, Berlin.

De Lacy, P. (trans.) (1996), *Galen: On the Elements According to Hippocrates*, Akademie Verlag, Berlin.

Diels, H. (ed.) (1915), *Galeni: In Hippocratis Prorrheticum I Commentaria Tria*, Akademie Verlag, Berlin.

Drabkin, I. (trans.) (1950), *Caelius Aurelius: On Acute and on Chronic Diseases*, University of Chicago Press, Chicago.

Forster, E.S. and Furley, D.J. (trans.) (1955), *Aristotle: On Sophistical Refutations, On Coming-to-be and Passing Away, On the Cosmos*, Cambridge, Massachusetts.

Fortuna, S. (1999), *A Patrofilo Sulla Constituzione Della Medicina*, Akademie Verlag GmbH, Berlin.

Fowler, H.N. (trans.) (1914), *Plato: Euthyphro, Apology, Crito, Phaedo, Phaedrus*, Cambridge, Massachusetts.

Fuchs, B. (trans.) and Garofalo, I. (ed.) (1997), *Anonymi Medici: De Morbis Acutis et Chroniis*, Brill, Leiden, New York, Köln.

Godley, A.D. (trans.) (1921), *Herodotus: The Persian Wars, Books 3–4*, Cambridge, Massachusetts.

Graham, D.W. (trans.) (2010), *The Texts of the Early Greek Philosophy: The Complete Fragments and Selected Testimonies of the Major Presocratics, Parts 1 and 2*, Cambrige: Cambridge University Press.

Grant, M. (trans.) (2000), *Galen on Food and Diet*, Routledge: London and New York.

Hankinson, R.J. (trans.) (1991), *Galen: On the Therapeutic Method, Books I and II*, Clarendon Press, Oxford.

Heeg, J. (ed.) (1915), *Galeni: In Hippocratis Prognosticum Commentaria Tria*, Akademie Verlag, Berlin.

Helmreich, G. (ed.) (1923), *Galeni: De Alimentorum Facultatibus*, Akademie Verlag, Berlin.

Helmreich, G. (ed.) (1914), *Galeni: In Hippocratis de Victu Acutorum Commentaria Quattuor*, Akademie Verlag, Berlin.

Hett, W.S. (trans.) (1957), *Aristotle: On the Soul, Parva Naturalia, On Breath*, Cambridge, Massachusetts.

Huffman, C.A. (trans.) (1993), *Philolaus of Croton: Pythagorean and Presocratic*, Cambridge University Press, Cambridge.

Johnston, I. (2006), *Galen on Diseases and Symptoms*, Cambridge University Press, Cambridge.

Jones, W.H.S. (trans.) (1923a), *Hippocrates: Volume I*, Cambridge, Massachusetts.

Jones, W.H.S. (trans.) (1923b), *Hippocrates: Volume II*, Cambridge, Massachusetts.

Jones, W.H.S. (trans.) (1931), *Hippocrates: Volume IV*, Cambridge, Massachusetts.

Jones, W.H.S. (trans.) (1947), *The Medical Writings of Anonymus Londinensis*, Cambridge University Press, Cambridge.

Jones, W.H.S. (trans.) (1956), *Pliny the Elder: Natural History, Books 24–27*, Cambridge, Massachusetts.

Jouanna, J. (2002a), *Hippocrate: La Nature de l'Homme*, Akademie Verlag, Berlin.

King, J.E. (trans.) (1927), *Cicero: Tusculan Disputations*, Cambridge, Massachusetts.

Kühn, C.G. (trans.) (2011), *Galeni Opera Omnia*, (20 vols. in 22), Leipzig (re-issued).

Lee, H.D.P. (trans.) (1952), *Aristotle: Meteorologica*, Cambridge, Massachusetts.

Littré, É. (trans.) (1961–1962), *Oeuvres Complètes d'Hippocrate, Tome première-neuvième*, Adolf M. Hakkert, Amsterdam.

Long, A.A. and Sedley, D.N., (trans.) (1987), *The Hellenistic Philosophers: Volume 1, Trans-*

lations of the Principal Sources, with Philosophical Commentary, Cambridge University Press, Cambridge.

Lonie, I.M. (trans.) (1981), *The Hippocratic treatises, "On generation," "On the nature of the child," "Diseases IV": a commentary*, Berlin; New York: De Gruyter.

May, M.T. (1968), *Galen: On the Usefulness of the Parts of the Body*, Cornell University Press, Ithaca New York.

Mayhew, R. (trans.) (2011), *Aristotle: Problems, Books 1–19, Rhetoric to Alexander*, Cambridge, Massachusetts.

Mayhew, R. and Mirhady, D.C. (trans.) (2011), *Aristotle: Problems, Books 20–38, Rhetoric to Alexander*, Cambridge, Massachusetts.

Mewaldt, I. (trans.) (1914), *Galeni: In Hippocratis de Natura Hominis Commentaria Tria*, Akademie Verlag, Berlin.

Murray, A.T. (trans.) and Wyatt, W.F. (rev.) (1925), *Homer: Iliad, Books 13–24*, Cambridge, Massachusetts.

Nickel, D. (trans.) (2001), *Galen: Über die Ausformung der Keimlinge*, Akademie Verlag, Berlin.

Nutton, V. (trans.) (1999), *Galen: On My Own Opinions*, Akademie Verlag, Berlin.

Peck, A.L. and Forster, E.S. (trans.) (1937), *Aristotle: Parts of Animals, Movement of Animals, Progression of Animals*, Cambridge, Massachusetts.

Peck, A.L. (trans.) (1965), *Aristotle: History of Animals, Books 1–3*, Cambridge, Massachusetts.

Pormann, P.E. (ed.) (2008), *Rufus of Ephesus, 'On Melancholy'*, Introduction, Text, Translation and Interpretative Essays, Tübingen.

Potter, P. (trans.) (1988a), *Hippocrates: Volume V*, Cambridge, Massachusetts.

Potter, P. (trans.) (1988b), *Hippocrates: Volume VI*, Cambridge, Massachusetts.

Potter, P. (trans.) (1995), *Hippocrates: Volume VIII*, Cambridge, Massachusetts.

Potter, P. (trans.) (2010), *Hippocrates: Volume IX*, Cambridge, Massachusetts.

Potter, P. (trans.) (2012), *Hippocrates: Volume X*, Cambridge, Massachusetts.

Singer, P. (trans.) (1997), *Galen: Selected Works*, Oxford World's Classics, Oxford.

Singer, P. (ed.) (2013), *Galen: Psychological Writings, Avoiding Distress Character Traits, The Diagnosis and Treatments of the Affections and Errors Peculiar to Each Person's Soul, the Capacities of the Soul Depend on the Mixtures of the Body*, Cambridge University Press, Cambridge.

Smith, C.F. (trans.) (1919), *Thucydides: History of the Peloponnesian War, Books 1–2*, Cambridge, Massachusetts.

Smith, W.D. (trans.) (1994), *Hippocrates: Volume VII*, Cambridge, Massachusetts.

Spencer, W.G. (trans.) (1935), *Celsus: On Medicine, Volume 1, Books 1–4*, Cambridge, Massachusetts.

Steckerl, F. (trans.) (1958), *The Fragments of Praxagoras of Cos and his School: Collected, Edited and Translated*, Brill, Leiden.

Van der Eijk, P.J. (trans.) (2000), *Diocles of Carystus: A Collection of the Fragments with Translation and Commentary, Volume 1: Text and Translation*, Brill, Leiden, Boston, Köln.

Van der Eijk, P.J. (trans.) (2001), *Diocles of Carystus: A Collection of the Fragments with Translation and Commentary, Volume 2: Commentary*, Brill, Leiden, Boston, Köln.

Van der Eijk, P.J. and Pormann, P.E. (trans.) (2008), 'Appendix 1: Greek Text, and Arabic and English Translations of Galen's *On the Affected Parts* iii. 9–10' in Pormann, P.E. (ed.), *Rufus of Ephesus, 'On Melancholy', Introduction, Text, Translation and Interpretative Essays*, Tübingen, pp. 265–287.

Von Staden, H. (trans.) (1989), *Herophilus: The Art of Medicine in Early Alexandria*, Cambridge University Press, Cambridge.

Wenkebach, E. (ed.) (1936), *Galeni: In Hippocratis Epidemiarum Librum III*, Akademie Verlag, Berlin.

Wenkebach, E. (ed.) and Pfaff, F. (trans.) (1934), *Galeni: In Hippocratis Epidemiarum Libros I et II*, Akademie Verlag, Berlin.

Wenkebach, E. (ed.) (1951), *Galeni: Adversus ea quae Iuliano In Hippocratis Aphorismos Enuntiata sunt Libellus*, Akademie Verlag, Berlin.

Wenkebach, E. (ed.) and Pfaff, F. (trans.) (1956), *Galeni: In Hippocratis Epidemiarum Librum VI Commentaria I–VIII*, Akademie Verlag, Berlin.

Wicksteed, P.H. and Cornford, F.M. (trans.) (1929), *Aristotle: Physics, Books I–IV*, Cambridge, Massachusetts.

Wilkins, J. (trans.) (2013), *Galien: Sur les Facultés des Aliments*, Les Belles Lettres, Paris.

Withington, E.T. (trans.) (2005), *Hippocrates: Volume III*, Cambridge, Massachusetts.

Secondary Sources

Arikha, N. (2007), *Passions and Tempers: A History of the Humours*, Harper Collins, New York.

Balme, D.M. (1987), 'Aristotle's Use of Division and Differentiae', in Gotthelf, A. and Lennox, J.G. (eds.), *Philosophical Issues in Aristotle's Biology*, Cambridge University Press, Cambridge, pp. 69–90.

Bell, M. (2014), *Melancholia: The Western Malady*, Cambridge University Press, Cambridge.

Bradley, M. (2009), *Colour and Meaning in Ancient Rome*, Cambridge University Press, Cambridge.

Chiaradonna, R., (2014), 'Galen on What is Persuasive (Pithanon) and What Approximates to Truth', in Adamson, P., Hansberger, R. and Wilberding, J. (eds.), *Philosophical Themes in Galen*, Institute of Classical Studies, School of Advanced Study, University of London, London, pp. 61–88.

Cornford, F.M. (1937), *Plato's Cosmology: The Timaeus of Plato translated with a running commentary*, Routledge, London.

Craik, E.M. (2015), *The Hippocratic Corpus: Content and Context*, Routledge, London and New York.

Deichgräber, K. (ed.) (1972), *Hippokrates' 'De humoribus' in der Geschichte der griechischen Medizin*, Akademie der Wissenschaften und der Literatur, Mainz, Abhandlungen der geistes- und sozialwissenschaftlichen Klasse XIV.

Demont, P. (2005), 'About Philosophy and Humoural Medicine', in van der Eijk, P.J. (ed.), *Hippocrates in Context: Papers Read at the XIth International Hippocrates Colloquium University of Newcastle upon Tyne 27–31*, Brill: Leiden and Boston, pp. 271–286.

Flashar, H. (1966), *Melancholie und Melancholiker in den medizinischen Theorien der Antike*, Berlin.

Flemming, R. (2008), 'Commentary', in Hankinson, R.J. (ed.), *The Cambridge Companion to Galen*, Cambridge University Press, Cambridge, pp. 323–354.

Flemming, R. (2009), 'Demiurge and Emperor in Galen's World of Knowledge', in Gill, C., Whitmarsh, T. and Wilkins, J. (eds.), *Galen and the World of Knowledge*, Cambridge University Press, Cambridge, pp. 59–84.

Frede, M. (1987), *Essays in Ancient Philosophy*, Clarendon Press, Oxford.

Furley, D.J. and Wilkie, J.S. (1984), *Galen on Respiration and the Arteries*, Princeton, New Jersey.

Garofalo, I. (2005), 'Galen's Commentary on Hippocrates' De humoribus', in van der Eijk, P.J., *Hippocrates in Context: Papers Read at the XIth International Hippocrates Colloquium University of Newcastle upon Tyne 27–31*, Brill: Leiden and Boston, pp. 445–456.

Gill, C. (2010), *Naturalistic Psychology in Galen and Stoicism*, Oxford: Oxford University Press.

Hankinson, R.J. (1992), 'Galen's Philosophical Eclecticism', in Haase, W. and Temporini, H. (eds.), *Aufstieg und Niedergang der römischen Welt*, De Gruyter, Berlin, pp. 3504–3522.

Hankinson, R.J. (1994a), 'Galen's Theory of Causation', in Haase, W. and Temporini, H. (eds.), *Aufstieg und Niedergang der römischen Welt*, De Gruyter, Berlin, pp. 1757–1774.

Hankinson, R.J. (1994b), 'Usage and Abusage: Galen on Language', in Everson, S. (ed.), *Philosophy of Language: Companions to Ancient Thought*, Vol. 3, Cambridge, pp. 166–193.

Hankinson, R.J. (2008), 'Philosophy of Nature', in Hankinson, R.J., *The Cambridge Companion to Galen*, Cambridge University Press, Cambridge, pp. 210–241.

Hankinson, R.J. (2009), 'Galen on the Limitations of Knowledge', in Gill, C., Whitmarsh, T. and Wilkins, J. (eds.), *Galen and the World of Knowledge*, Cambridge University Press, Cambridge, pp. 206–242.

Hanson, A.E. (1998), 'Galen: Author and Critic', in Most, G.W. (ed.), *Editing Texts: Texte edieren*, Gottingen, pp. 22–53.

Harig, G. and Kollesch, J. (1975), 'Galen und Hippokrates' in *La Collection Hippocratique et son Role dans l'Histoire de la Medicine*, Leiden, Brill, pp. 257–274.

Harris, W.V. (2013), 'Thinking about Mental Disorders in Classical Antiquity' in Harris, W.V. (ed.), *Mental Disorders in the Classical World*, Brill, Leiden and Boston, pp. 1–26.

Jouanna, J. (2001), *Hippocrates*, Johns Hopkins University Press, Baltimore and London.

Jouanna, J. (2002b), 'La notion de nature chez Galien', in Barnes, J. and Jouanna, J. (eds.), *Galien et la Philosophie*, Vandoeuvres, Genève, pp. 229–268.

Jouanna, J. (2006), 'La postérité du traité Hippocratique de la Nature de l'homme: la théorie des quatre humeurs', in Müller, C.W., Brockmann, C. and Brunschön, C.W. (eds), *Arzte und ihre Interpreten*, Leipzig: Saur, pp. 117–141.

Jouanna, J. (2009), 'Bile noire et mélancholie chez Galien: le traité sur la bile noire est-il authentique?', in Brockmann, C., Brunschön, C.W., Overwien, O. (eds.), *Antike Medizin in Schnittpunkt von Geistes- und Naturwissenschaften. Internationale Fachtagung aus Anlass des 100 jährigen Vestehens des Akademievorhabens "Corpus Medicorum Graecorum Latinorum"*, Müchen and Leipzig, pp. 235–257.

Jouanna, J. (2012a), 'At the Roots of Melancholy: Is Greek Medicine Melancholic?' in van der Eijk (ed.) and Allies, N. (trans.), *Greek Medicine from Hippocrates to Galen: Selected Papers by Jacques Jouanna*, Brill, Leiden and Boston, pp. 229–258.

Jouanna, J. (2012b), 'Galen's Reading of the Hippocratic Treatise *The Nature of Man*: The Foundations of Hippocratism in Galen' in van der Eijk (ed.) and Allies, N. (trans.), *Greek Medicine from Hippocrates to Galen: Selected Papers by Jacques Jouanna*, Brill, Leiden and Boston, pp. 313–333.

Kazantzidis, G. (2013), '*Quem nos furorem, μελαγχολίαν illi vocant*: Cicero on Melancholy' in Harris, W.V. (ed.), *Mental Disorders in the Classical World*, Brill, Leiden and Boston, pp. 245–264.

Klibansky, R., Panofsky, E. and Saxl, F. (1964), *Saturn and Melancholy: Studies in the History of Natural Philosophy, Religion and Art*, Nelson: London.

Kudlien, F. (1964a), 'Bakcheios', *Der kleine Pauly* 1: col. 808.

Kudlien, F. (1964b), 'Herophilus und der Beginn der medizinischen Skepsis', *Gesnerus* 21, pp. 1–13.

Kupreeva, I., (2014), 'Galen's Theory of Elements', in Adamson, P., Hansberger, R. and Wilberding, J. (eds.), *Philosophical Themes in Galen*, Institute of Classical Studies, School of Advanced Study, University of London, London, pp. 153–196.

Langholf, V., (1990), *Medical theories in Hippocrates: early texts and the "Epidemics"*, Walter de Gruyter, Berlin.

Leith, D.L. (2009), 'The Qualitative Status of the *onkoi* in Asclepiades' Theory of Matter', *Oxford Studies in Ancient Philosophy*, 36, pp. 283–320.

Leith, D.L. (2012), 'Pores and Void in Asclepiades' Physical Theory', *Phronesis*, 57, pp. 164–191.

Leith, D.L., (2014), 'Galen's Refutation of Atomism', in Adamson, P., Hansberger, R. and

Wilberding, J. (eds.), *Philosophical Themes in Galen*, Institute of Classical Studies, School of Advanced Study, University of London, London, pp. 213–234.

Leith, D.L. (2015a), 'Elements and Uniform Parts in Early Alexandrian Medicine', *Phronesis*, 60, Brill, pp. 462–491.

Leith, D.L. (2015b), 'Erasistratus' *Triplokia* of Arteries, Veins and Nerves', *apeiron*, 48(3), De Gruyter, pp. 251–262.

Leith, D.L. (Forthcoming), 'Asclepiades of Bithynia as Hippocratic Commentator', pp. 1–17.

Liddell, H.G., Scott, R. (eds.) and Jones, H.S. (rev.) (1940) *A Greek-English Lexicon*, Clarendon Press, Oxford.

Lloyd, G.E.R. (1963), 'Who is attacked in *On Ancient Medicine*', *Pronesis* 8, pp. 108–126.

Lloyd, G.E.R. (1975), 'The Hippocratic Question', *The Classical Quarterly*, Vol. 25, Issue 02 (December), pp. 171–192.

Lloyd, G.E.R. (1993), 'Galen on Hellenistics and Hippocrateans: Contemporary Battles and Past Authorities' in Kollesch, J. and Nickel, D., *Galen und das Hellenistic Erbe*, Franz Steiner Verlag, Stuttgart, pp. 125–144.

Lloyd, G.E.R. (1996), 'Theories and Practices of Demonstration in Galen', in Frede, M. and Striker, G. (eds.), *Rationality in Greek Thought*, Clarendon Press, Oxford, pp. 255–277.

Lloyd, G.E.R. (2003), *In the Grip of Disease: Studies in the Greek Imagination*, Oxford University Press, Oxford.

Lloyd, G.E.R. (2008), 'Galen and his Contemporaries', *Cambridge Companion to Galen*, Cambridge University Press, Cambridge, pp. 34–48.

Magner, L.N. (1992), *A History of Medicine*, Marcel Dekker Inc., New York and Basel.

Manetti, D. and Roselli, A. (1994), 'Galeno commentatore di Ippocrate', *ANRW*, II 37.2, pp. 1529–1635.

Manetti, D. (1999), 'Aristotle and the Role of Doxography in the Anonymus Londinensis (PbrLibr Inv. 137)', in van der Eijk, P.J. (ed.), *Ancient Histories of Medicine: Essays in Medical Doxography and Historiography in Classical Antiquity*, Brill, Leiden, Boston and Köln, pp. 95–142.

Manetti, D. (2009), 'Galen and Hippocratic Medicine: language and practice', in Gill, C., Whitmarsh, T. and Wilkins, J. (eds.), *Galen and the World of Knowledge*, Cambridge University Press, Cambridge, pp. 157–174.

Mattern, S.P. (2008), *Galen & the Rhetoric of Healing*, The John Hopkins University Press, Baltimore.

Mattern, S.P. (2013), *The Prince of Medicine: Galen in the Roman Empire*, Oxford University Press, Oxford.

Morison, B. (2008), 'Logic', in Hankinson, R.J., *The Cambridge Companion to Galen*, Cambridge University Press, Cambridge, pp. 66–115.

Müri, W. (1953), "Melancholie und schwarze Galle", *Museum Helveticum* 10, pp. 21–38.

Nutton, V. (2004), *Ancient Medicine*, London.

Nutton, V. (2005), 'The Fatal Embrace: Galen and the History of Ancient Medicine', *Science in Context*, 18(1), pp. 111–121.

Nutton, V. (2013), 'Galenic Madness' in Harris, W.V. (ed.), *Mental Disorders in the Classical World*, Brill, Leiden and Boston, pp. 119–128.

Pellegrin, P. (2009), 'Ancient Medicine and its Contribution to the Philosophical Tradition', in Gill, M.L. and Pellegrin, P., *A Companion to Ancient Philosophy*, Wiley-Blackwell, Chichester UK, pp. 664–684.

Pendrick, G. (1994), 'A Note on Galen and Asclepiades', *Mnemosyne*, Fourth Series, Vol. 47, Fasc. 2, pp. 226–229.

Pigeaud, J. (1980), 'La physiologie de Lucrèce' ['Physiologie'], *Revues des études latines*, 58, pp. 176–200.

Pigeaud, J. (1981), *La maladie de l'ame. Etude sur la relation de l'âme et du corps dans la tradition medico-philosophique antique*, Paris.

Polito, R. (2006), 'Matter, Medicine, and the Mind: Asclepiades vs. Epicurus', *Oxford Studies in Ancient Philosophy*, 30, pp. 285–335.

Pormann, P.E. (2013), 'Medical Epistemology and Melancholy: Rufus of Ephesus and Miskawayh' in Harris, W.V. (ed.), *Mental Disorders in the Classical World*, Brill, Leiden and Boston, pp. 223–244.

Porter, R. (1997), *The Greatest Benefit to Mankind: A Medical History of Humanity from Antiquity to the Present*, Fontana Press, London.

Porter, R. (2003), *Blood and Guts: A Short History of Medicine*, London: Penguin Books.

Roselli, A. (1999), 'The *Doxai* of Doctors in Galen's Commentaries', in van der Eijk, P.J. (ed.), *Ancient Histories of Medicine: Essays in Medical Doxography and Historiography in Classical Antiquity*, Brill, Leiden, Boston, Köln, pp. 359–381.

Roselli, A. (2015), 'Galeno sull'autenticità del Prorretico I', in Holmes, B. and Fischer, K.-D. (eds.), *The Frontiers of Ancient Science: Essays in Honour of Heinrich von Staden*, de Gruyter, Berlin, pp. 533–559.

Schiefsky, M. (2007), 'Galen's Teleology and Functional Explanations' in Sedley, D. (ed.), *Oxford Studies in Ancient Philosophy*, Oxford University Press, Oxford, pp. 369–400.

Schöner, E. (1964), *Das Viererschema in der antiken Humoralpathologie*, Wiesbaden (Sudhoffs Archiv, Beih. 4).

Schütrumpf, E. (2015), 'Black bile as the Cause of Human Accomplishments and Behaviors in *Pr.* 30.1: Is the Concept Aristotelian?' in Mayhew, R. (ed.), *The Aristotelian "Problemata Physica", Philosophical and Scientific Investigations*, Brill, Leiden, Boston, pp. 357–380.

Seale, C. (1994), 'Health and Healing in an Age of Science', in Seale, C. and Pattison, S., *Medical Knowledge: Doubt and Certainty*, The Open University Press, Buckingham, pp. 7–27.

Sharples, R.W. (1995), *Theophrastus of Eresus: Sources for his Life, Writings, Thought and*

Influence: Commentary Volume 5, Sources of Biology (Human Physiology, Living Creatures, Botany: Texts 328–435), Brill, Leiden, Boston, Köln.

Sharples, R.W. (1998), *Theophrastus of Eresus: Sources for his Life, Writings, Thought and Influence: Commentary Volume 3.1, Sources of Physics (Texts 137–223)*, Brill, Leiden, Boston, Köln.

Siegel, R.E. (1968), *Galen's System of Physiology and Medicine*, Basle, New York.

Singer, P.N., (2014), 'Galen and the Philosophers: Philosophical Engagement, Shadowy Contemporaries, Aristotelian Transformations', in Adamson, P., Hansberger, R. and Wilberding, J. (eds.), *Philosophical Themes in Galen*, Institute of Classical Studies, School of Advanced Study, University of London, London, pp. 7–38.

Sluiter, I. (1995), 'The Embarrassment of Imperfection: Galen's Assessment of Hippocrates' Linguistic Merits', in van der Eijk, P.J., Horstmanshoff, H. f. J. and Schrijvers, P.H. (eds.), *Ancient Medicine in its Socio-Cultural Context: Papers read at the congress held at Leiden University, 13–15 April 1992, Volume II*, Amsterdam—Atlanta, GA, pp. 519–535.

Small, P.J. (1997), *Wax Tablets of the Mind: Cognitive Studies of Memory and Literacy in Classical Antiquity*, London and New York.

Smith, W.D. (1979), *The Hippocratic Tradition*, Cornell University Press, Ithaca and London.

Swain, S. (1996), *Hellenism and Empire: Language, Classicism and Power in the Greek World A D 50–250*, Clarendon Press, Oxford.

Thomas, O. (2015), 'Creating *Problemata* with the Hippocratic Corpus' in Mayhew, R. (ed.), *The Aristotelian "Problemata Physica", Philosophical and Scientific Investigations*, Brill, Leiden and Boston, pp. 79–99.

Vallance, J.T. (1990), *The Lost Theory of Asclepiades of Bithynia*, Clarendon, Oxford.

Vallance, J.T. (2000), 'Doctors in the Library: The Strange Tale of Apollonius the Bookworm and Other Stories', in MacLeod, R. (ed.), *The Library of Alexandria: Centre of Learning in the Ancient World*, London and New York, pp. 95–113.

van der Eijk, P.J. (1999), 'Historical Awareness, Historiography, and Doxography in Greek and Roman Medicine', in van der Eijk, P.J. (ed.), *Ancient Histories of Medicine: Essays in Medical Doxography and Historiography in Classical Antiquity*, Brill, Leiden, Boston, Köln, pp. 1–31.

van der Eijk, P.J. (2005), *Medicine and Philosophy in Classical Antiquity: Doctors and Philosophers on Nature, Soul, Health and Disease*, Cambridge University Press, Cambridge.

van der Eijk, P.J. (2012), 'Aristotle! What a Thing for You to Say!' in Gill, C., Whitmarsh, T. and Wilkins, J. (eds.), *Galen and the World of Knowledge*, Cambridge University Press, Cambridge, pp. 261–281.

van der Eijk, P.J. (2014), 'Galen on the Nature of Human Beings', in Adamson, P., Hansberger, R. and Wilberding, J. (eds.), *Philosophical Themes in Galen*, Institute of Classical Studies, School of Advanced Study, University of London, London, pp. 89–134.

Vegetti, M. (1999a), 'Tradition and truth. Forms of philosophical-scientific historiography in Galen's *De Placitis*' in van der Eijk, P.J. (ed.), *Ancient Histories of Medicine: Essays in Medical Doxography and Historiography in Classical Antiquity*, Brill, Leiden, Boston, Köln, pp. 333–358.

Vegetti, M. (1999b), 'Historical strategies in Galen's physiology' in van der Eijk, P.J. (ed.), *Ancient Histories of Medicine: Essays in Medical Doxography and Historiography in Classical Antiquity*, Brill, Leiden, Boston, Köln, pp. 383–395.

von Staden, H. (1982), 'Hairesis and Heresy: The Case of the Haireseis Iatrikai', in Meyer, B.F. and Sanders, E.P. (eds.), *Jewish and Christian Self-Definition, Volume 3: Self-Definition in the Graeco-Roman World*, SCM Press Ltd, London, pp. 76–100.

von Staden, H. (1995), 'Science as text, science as history: Galen on metaphor', in van der Eijk, P.J., Horstmanshoff, J.F.J. and Schrijvers, P.H. (eds.), *Ancient Medicine in its Socio-Cultural Context: Papers read at the congress held at Leiden University, 13–15 April 1992, Volume II*, Amsterdam—Atlanta, GA, pp. 499–518.

von Staden, H. (1997a), 'Galen and the "Second Sophistic"', *Bulletin of the Institute of Classical Studies*, Vol. 41, Issue S68 (January), pp. 33–54.

von Staden, H. (1997b), 'Teleology and Mechanism: Aristotelian Biology and Early Hellenic Medicine', in Kullman, W. and Föllinger, S. (eds.), *Aristotelische Biologie, Intentionen, Ergeb*, Steiner, Stuttgart, pp. 183–208.

von Staden, H. (1999a), 'Rupture and Continuity: Hellenistic Reflections on the History of Medicine', in van der Eijk, P.J. (ed.), *Ancient Histories of Medicine: Essays in Medical Doxography and Historiography in Classical Antiquity*, Brill, Leiden, Boston, Köln, pp. 143–187.

von Staden, H. (1999b), 'Celsus as Historian?', in van der Eijk, P.J. (ed.), *Ancient Histories of Medicine: Essays in Medical Doxography and Historiography in Classical Antiquity*, Brill, Leiden, Boston, Köln, pp. 251–294.

von Staden, (2006a), 'Interpreting 'Hippokrates' in the 3rd and 2nd Centuries BC', in Müller, C.W., Brockmann, C. and Brunschön, C.W. (eds.), *Ärzte und ihre Interpreten: Medizinische Fachtexte der Antike als Forschungsgegenstand der Klassischen Philologie*, K.G. Saur München, Leipzig, pp. 15–47.

von Staden, (2006b), 'Staging the Past, Staging Oneself: Galen on Hellenistic Exegetical Traditions', in Gill, C., Whitmarsh, T. and Wilkins, J. (eds.), *Galen and the World of Knowledge*, Cambridge University Press, Cambridge, pp. 132–156.

Wellmann, M. (1895), *Die Pneumatische Schule bis auf Archigenes*, Weidmannsche Buchhandlung, Berlin.

Index

Index of Sources

Printed in the United States
by Baker & Taylor Publisher Services